Unsung Stories of
Covid 19 & Lockdown

Unsung Stories of
Covid 19 & Lockdown

Kumar Shyam

YASH PUBLICATIONS
Delhi-110032

Unsung Stories of Covid 19 & Lockdown

ISBN : 978-93-81130-40-7

First Edition : October : 2020

These stories are inspired by recent events. However, they are purely works of fiction. Names, characters, businesses, places, events and incidents are either the products of the author's imagination or used in a fictitious manner. Any resemblance to actual persons, living or dead, is purely coincidental.

Published by : Yash Publications
1/10753, Subhash Park, Naveen Shahdara
Delhi-110032 (India)

Sales Office : 4754/23, Ansari Road,
Daryaganj, New Delhi-110002

Helpline : +011-40018100
E-mail: sales@yashpublications.co.in
Website: www.yashpublications.co.in
e-book avilable at : *amazon.in, flipkart.com*

“There are only two ways to live your life. One is as though nothing is a miracle. The other is as though everything is a miracle.”

– Albert Einstein

Contents

Preface

There are some years in every person's life which change his/her perspective towards life itself. 2020 has been such a year for not just one person but perhaps the entire human race. The Covid-19 pandemic is an event that none of us had witnessed before, and I pray to the Almighty that we never see a repeat of it in our lives. We can think of it as a wake-up call, teaching us how to treat Mother Nature, and to remind us that despite our scientific achievements we are still a part of the natural ecosystem and not its master.

Just like any other crisis, the COVID-19 outbreak, while it has caused great suffering and loss to human life, has also brought forth some of the most extraordinary demonstrations of love and empathy by human beings towards one another.

This collection of stories was inspired by some of these displays of resilience and the unbreakable human spirit, which I have tried to capture using my imagination.

This is a kind of my tribute to all those who suffered during the pandemic, and to those who fought bravely to alleviate the sufferings of others in these adverse times.

The other stories too are narrated from the events happening in our surroundings to explore different human emotions and behaviour.

Kumar Shyam

ACKNOWLEDGEMENT

This book is a culmination of not only of my efforts but those of multiple people. They include my daughter Himani, who gave the characters in the stories a face with her illustrations; my son Devesh, who gave his valuable feedback; my younger son Abhidev, who wrote two of the stories and graciously offered to share them in this book.

A special thank to Dr. Govind Singh, Dr. Vimlesh Sharma and Dr. Shiv Kumar who are always my back bone.

A special note of thanks to my wife Santosh, who, for all these days bear with me, and my busy schedule.

I would like to thank Dr. Sanjay Rai, Nipunika, Niharika and all my colleagues who encourged me to pen down the stories.

Another note of thanks is to my nephews – Neeraj, Sandeep and Himanshu – who helped in reviewing and structuring the stories.

I would also like to acknowledge Debashish Mukherji for his help in the final editing and structuring of the stories.

A last special thanks to Puneet Sharma and Yash Publications who made it possible to bring this book to a larger reader base.

THE SUDDEN SHOCK

"Has papa become an untouchable now?" Five years old Bunty asked his mother.

His father, Dr Dinesh Khatri was a Civil Surgeon and in-charge of the COVID-19 unit at Government hospital. After five days of continuous duty he had returned home. He was sitting on a cemented edge outside the main gate of his house alongside the driveway. Bunty, ecstatic at seeing his father after five long days, ran to hug him. But the main gate, still shut, was in his way. He expected his father to open the gate and pick him as he usually did.

But his expectations were shattered. His father remained seated where he was. Bunty was confused. His mother came out behind him, but she too did not open the gate – all she did was smile at his father. Their two year old Labrador golden retriever, Tyson, who had been with the family since he was eight days old, kept barking madly. Bunty's mother asked Tyson and Bunty to calm down. But neither of them seemed to listen.

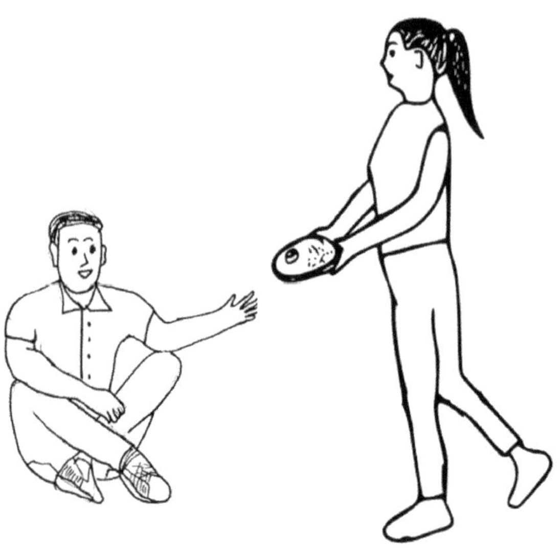

She went back inside, and returned to the main gate of their bungalow with food and a glass of water. But she still did not open the gate. Dr. Khatri stepped forward to take the food and ate it still sitting outside the house. Dr. Khatri gazed at his family with love. He returned the empty plate and glass to his wife. A tear trickled down his cheek as he walked back to his car. He started his car and went back to the hospital with a heavy heart.

Bunty and Tyson stared at the car until it was out of sight. Then Bunty sobbed with arms outstretched. He was unable to understand and approached his mother, as she was putting the plate and glass used by his father in a separate corner, away from other used utensils.

Has papa become an untouchable now? Bunty asked again.

“No, but why do you ask?” His mother replied.

“Mom, I have seen the same practice in a serial based on Dr. Ambedkar. The untouchables were not allowed to enter the house.”

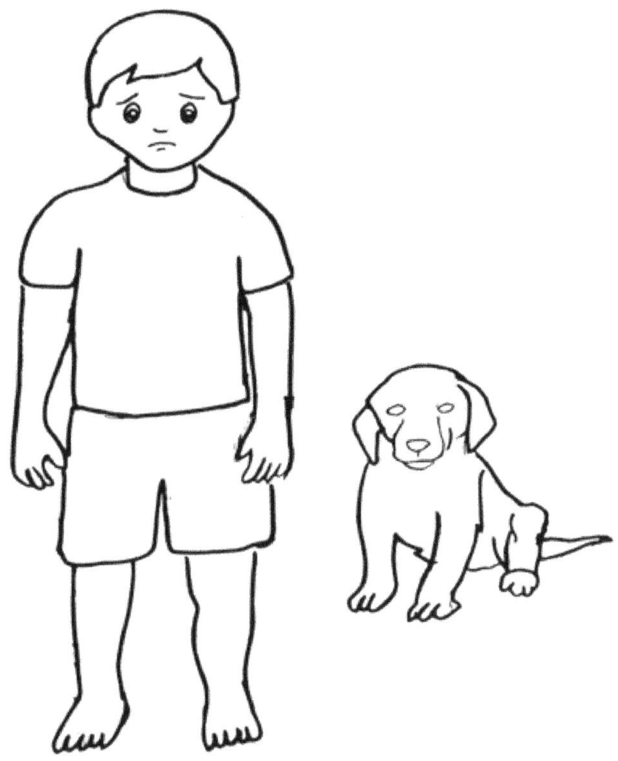

Shocked and stunned she raised Bunty in her arms and replied.

“No son, you will understand it later,”.

Bunty was not at all convinced, but he went away to play with Tyson.

"What mom said is not true. I am sure that papa is an untouchable now," he complained to Tyson.

Tyson wagged his tail and licked Bunty's face.

COVID -19, Making a new class of Untouchables.

Untouchability is worst social evil, Forbidden and Unlawful.

ATHEIST VS. THEIST

Vimlesh looked at the alarm clock by her bedside. It was 5.00 am, her usual time to wake up. She no longer needed an alarm to wake at this time. She moved the curtains aside to look outside. It was still dark but soon the dark shades of the night would be replaced by the golden rays of a new day. She had always felt early morning to be the most positive time of the day.

She had wonderful flowers and precious plants in her terrace garden. There were often house birds' there – sparrows, koels, kingfishers and doves. Pigeons lived there like permanent residents. It was her routine, for the past 12 years, to place grains for the birds and water the plants before sunrise. The birds had gotten friendly; they were so familiar with her presence and her being punctual that they would start making a noise if she was late by even a few minutes.

Chunnu was Vimlesh's eldest daughter, studying for her graduation. Unlike Vimlesh, who was very religious, Chunnu maintained she was an atheist. That morning, Vimlesh was startled to find Chunnu had woken up before her, and was praying "What a great surprise, Chunnu is a believer now!" Vimlesh thought. She wondered if she was dreaming.

Chunnu never entered temples or shrines. She would always sit outside temple complexes, while others went in, saying she would take care of their footwear, which they would take off before entering.

Stealing of shoes from outside temples and shrines is a normal thing in many places in India. Many people visit temples deliberately wearing old, ragged footwear, which they quietly exchange with new ones taken off by other visitors who are still inside. Indeed, devotees at temples, seeking blessings and luck, often don't mind losing their shoes or sandals, considering the loss part of their temple offering and being used by someone in need. There was a man who boasted in his old age that in all his life of six decades he never spent a single paisa on shoes and yet always had dozens of branded shoes.

"Chunnu, are you okay," Vimlesh finally asked.

"Yes, mom."

"Today the sun seems to be rising from the west," Vimlesh smiled and said

"The sun is rising from the east as always," Chunnu smiled and answered. "I have discovered God."

"You discovered God? That's great, my dear. I know you never visited any temple, shrine or church," Vimlesh said, smiling sardonically.

"Mom, I have always paid my respects to temples and shown my regard for them. I have always appreciated the beautiful, mesmerizing architecture of all places of God. Do you remember, I visited Akshardham and Birla Mandir in Delhi and Meenakshipuram Temple in Madurai?"

While sitting outside the temples?" Vimlesh asked.

"I was taking care of the shoes, mom."

"At every shrine you went to?"

"Yes of course, everywhere."

"But many of those places already had people assigned to safeguard devotees' shoes."

"Yes, Mom, but remember you said many times that God is everywhere. So, what's the difference if I am inside or outside a shrine?"

Vimlesh wasn't prepared for such debate early in the morning. She couldn't counter Chunnu's argument. "Chunnu is anyway right. God is everywhere," she thought.

"Mom, is God visible?" Chunnu asked.

"No, God is invisible."

"Do we need to be afraid of God?"

"Yes, everyone should be afraid of God."

"Mom, have you ever seen God? You have been visiting temples and shrines for almost four decades."

"No, my child, never."

"Mom, why are you not going to the temple nowadays?"

"Temples are closed, Chunnu, don't you know that!"

"And what about, mosques, churches, gurudwaras, and other shrines?"

"They are all closed, my child. We are told about it daily by newspapers and news channels."

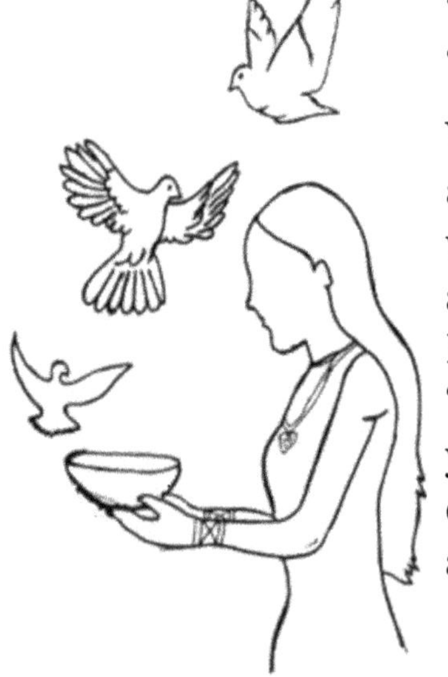

"Why, mom?"

Vimlesh was surprised again – how could her will aware daughter ask such a question? But she answered it. "It's the fear of corona, you know. Social distancing is a must, and advisable."

"Mom can you see this corona?"

"No."

"Mom, you are a doctor, can you treat it?"

"No, there is no treatment yet."

"You are also afraid of it?"

"Yes."

"Is it here in India only?

"No, it's a pandemic, it's all over the world."

"Can any divine power save us from the corona?"

"No."

"Mom, temples are closed, mosques are closed, churches are closed, and all other shrines are closed. Every public place in the world is closed. Roads are deserted, trains don't move, and planes are grounded no-one is allowed to move freely. Poor or rich, Hindu or Muslim, Buddhist or Christian, theist or atheist, everyone on the planet is afraid. East or west, north or south, there is fear only. The Fear of death." She took a deep breath.

"Yes, unfortunately, that is correct," Vimlesh agreed.

"So mom, I decided to pray to the one which has created this fear and compelled every one to shut all doors to the God.

"Means?" Vimlesh was confused.

"Mom it's the fear of the unseen, the fear of losing something, fear of death that compels people to bow down to an invisible power they call God. But at this moment, this unseen power is corona and there is absolutely nothing to save us from this pandemic no doctors, no medicines etc. I was an atheist but now I am a theist. After all, it's a matter of life, mom. Corona Dev, have mercy on us."

Vimlesh stood speechless. She didn't know how long she stood still, thinking about what Chunnu had just said. Her trance was broken by the commotion of the birds waiting for the grains.

"Are you not afraid of corona?" she asked the birds.

> It is better to be an outspoken atheist than a hypocrite.
>
> "George Harrison"

The Declaration at 8PM

"Take it," said Geeta handing over a briefcase to Sanjay.

"What is this?" He was confused.

"You were asking for money one week back. Here it is," she replied.

"Oh yes, I needed it that time. But you had said that you didn't have any, so I took a loan from a friend," said Sanjay. He was still confused.

Sanjay had been in dire need of money a week ago. He knew that Geeta saved a lot from the money he handed her every month for household expenses.

But it was only two and a half years ago that he realized how much she used to save. At the time of demonetization she had given him Rs 650,000 (6.5 lac). On 8th November 2017, to everybody's surprise, the Prime Minister had declared that from 12pm that night, 500 rupees and 1000-rupees notes would not remain to be legal tenders anymore.

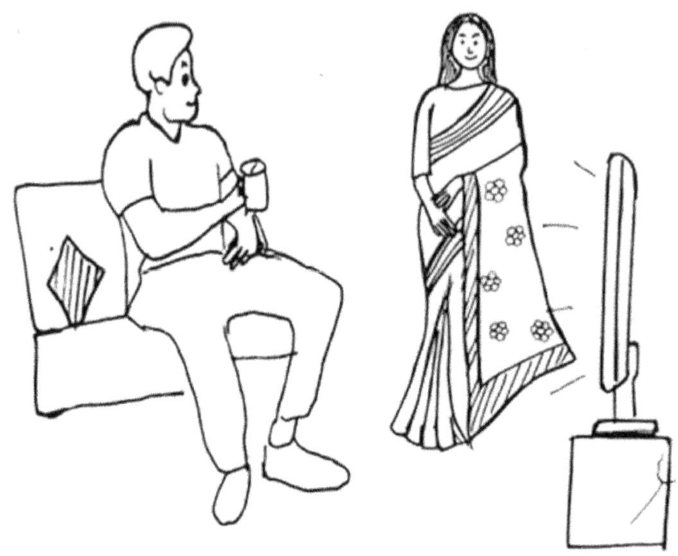

Sanjay wasn't much bothered by the announcement as his savings were in bank deposits. But Geeta was shocked. She felt that the Prime Minister had raided her faith and her hard-earned treasure, despite her having been his blind follower (or a bhakt, as many people call such followers.) But from then on, the Prime Minister had become the biggest villain in her eyes. On the other hand, Sanjay became his biggest fan as he received the hidden treasure.

Cut to the present. "How much is it?"Sanjay asked as he opened the briefcase.

"Not much it is only Rs 11000,00, (11 lac) consisting of Rs 2000 notes. Actually, I just forgot that I had this," she lied with a straight face.

"Okay. I will repay the loan with this," Sanjay said, putting the briefcase aside and opening a bottle of Jack Daniel. He didn't believe Geeta's statement about having forgotten the money, but said nothing. After 14 years of marriage, he had learned when to keep his mouth shut.

"You are a saviour, my dear," he said, wondering about Geeta's sudden change of attitude.

Unable to comprehend it, he focused on his favorite whisky. Geeta got busy in the kitchen preparing dinner.

Sanjay kept on enjoying his whisky. He was watching a news channel. Suddenly the channel announced the prime minister was going to address the country at 8 pm.

"Maybe it is some statement on the Citizenship Act or the National Population Register," he thought. Both had been subjects of much controversy recently. There had been processions and dharnas against them in many places. The dharnas at Shaheen Bagh and Jamia Millia University in Delhi were, in particular, attracting national and international media attention. In a few places, the processions opposing the government had become violent too.

Soon it was 8pm. Sanjay took the remote and raised the volume of his 42-inch flat screen TV. Geeta also joined him to watch.

"My dear countrymen, from tonight 12pm onwards........"

"…. the 2000 rupee note will not be a legal tender" Geeta thought.

Sanjay was expecting to hear something about the Citizenship Act or the NPR.

.... the country will be in lockdown," the Prime Minister completed his sentence.

The Prime Minister continued, "My dear countrymen, consider it an emergency. It's for you and your loved ones. The danger of Covid-19 infecting you is paramount. All of you should stay where you are. Emergency services will continue as they are. Wear masks, wash your hands repeatedly, use hand sanitizer and keep distance from one another."

"Give me my bag, my money." Geeta literally snatched the briefcase from Sanjay's side.

Her Prime Minster had not ditched her this time. Her money was safe.

Sanjay was shocked. There were hardly a handful of cases of corona in India. Why this step? He was unhappy. He gave the briefcase with its Rs 11000,00, (11 lac) back to his wife with a heavy heart. Now he understood the reason behind the sudden spark of philanthropy in his wife's heart.

The spark which had kindled abruptly had also been extinguished just as abruptly.

Geeta was happy. She waited for him to join her for dinner. She had cooked his favorite dishes.

"Keep your distance from me, Corona is here," he said to Geeta and asked her to obey the words of the Prime Minister. He took two more pegs of Jack Daniel and passed out in his chair.

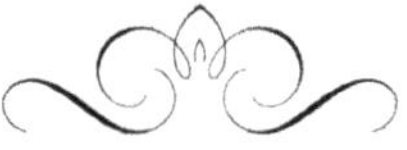

> We have to distruct each other, it is our only defense against betrayal.
>
> "Tennessee Williams"

New York – A City of The Deads

"Forty five year old male, University Professor, run over by a car near the exit from the southern highway towards downtown, extensive blood loss, multiple fractures and low pulse," a voice shattered the radio silence of an NYPD patrol car.

This was the man Trevor Laddy the acused who had hit the Professor Daniel Lewis to take revenge, on failing his girlfriend Delphine in her University exams. Trevor didn't care much whether Delphine passed or failed the exam, but her result impacted his future. Her father had set one condition for their marriage – she had to complete her education. He couldn't bear to wait another year for her to marry him. He had intended to just frighten the professor. But in his intoxicated state, he had gone too far. And now it had been 10 years that Trevor had been in Rikers Island prison, sentenced to life imprisonment for murder and reckless driving.

Still, he had a good rapport with jailor Stephen Smith. They often went with other prisoners to Hart Island where the prisoners dug graves for unclaimed dead bodies.

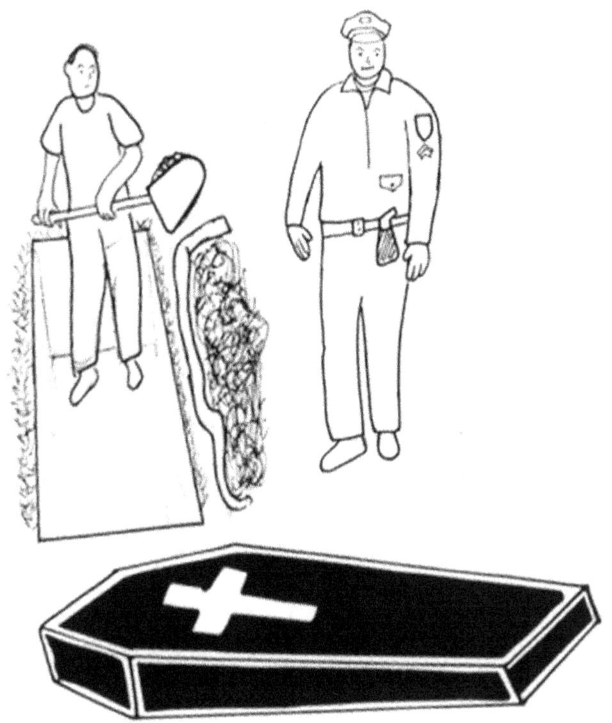

SCENE: Trevor is digging, with Stephen sitting on a rock nearby.

TREVOR: Another fine day, isn't it?

(Stephen nods)

TREVOR: You are one of the few good people I know. I would gladly dig a grave just like this for you with no hard feelings.

(Stephen gives him a hard look.)

TREVOR: Sorry, I was just kidding.

(Stephen laughs and Trevor joins him too.)

TREVOR: I was also a good person like you once.

STEPHEN: Is that so?

TREVOR: Back in my golden days, I had everything one could fancy. You know the typical New Yorker's life. Spending time with my loved ones, going shopping in Behemoth Shopping Complexes and malls in Times Square, going for late night walks on the streets, visiting the libraries, the museums... I did it all. I just love NYC, it has everything. You just name it. There is nothing in the world that NYC cannot give you. Life was bright back then until... you know how I ended up here.

STEPHEN: Sorry to hear that. But it's not just you who misses his life. The corona virus has taken away from New Yorkers, all the joy and liveliness the city gave them.

TREVOR: You must have been to the city. What is the scene like in the city?

STEPHEN: It is totally different from what we used to see. The city is completely silent, no musicians on the streets, no artists performing, no rumble of high-end sports cars. The city looks lonely with hardly its people being visible. And for the first time in history the land seems clearer than the sky.

TREVOR: It must be hard for you to see that every day.

STEPHEN: It is, really. People are baffled and scared. Ambulances roar down the streets like lions and make people around wonder if they might be the next prey. The ambulances are the kings of the street now.

TREVOR: I cannot imagine how people must be feeling.

STEPHEN: I'm not sure if the city even recovered from the 9/11 attack. And now, this corona has come to take away what was left. I pity the people and their pain.

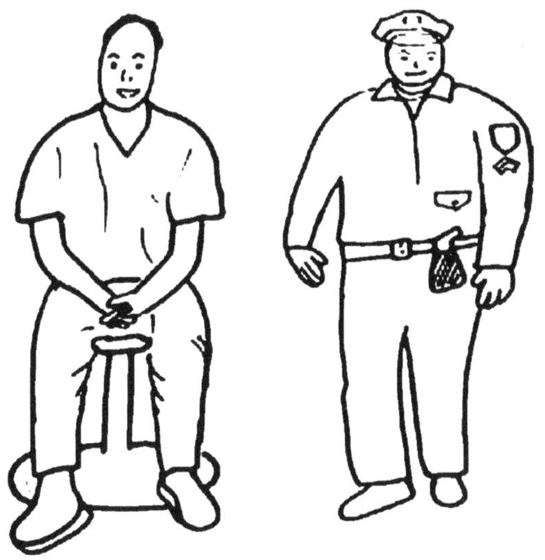

TREVOR: The city seems to have lost its life.

STEPHEN: It has. The city, the pride of America, seems to be dead now.

TREVOR: The sound of that makes even the prison seems better.

STEPHEN: (with a grin) Sure does.

TREVOR: Though not all people are infected by the virus, it seems to have infected everybody's life.

STEPHEN: Sounds about right.

TREVOR: Speak... (pauses as he covers his mouth to cough)....speaking of the city, it is an alpha++ rated city, isn't it?

STEPHEN: Yeah.

TREVOR: Isn't it strange that such a city could be so hard hit by COVID-19?

STEPHEN: Not really, because it's one of the most visited cities in the world, and that has spread the virus.

TREVOR: That makes sense.

The two men talk until it is time to pack up.

STEPHEN: Good job today.

(The two men shake hands)

The next day saw no activity when it was time to go to Hart Island again. Trevor asked Stephen why.

TREVOR: Aren't we supposed to go to the Island?

STEPHEN: We were. But orders came from above to immediately stop the grave preparing work the prisoners were doing. It is being handed over to commercial contractors due to the COVID-19 outbreak and tremendous rise in casualties.

TREVOR: Casualties? How many?

STEPHEN: In hundreds, maybe 700 plus per day, if you believe the newspapers.

TREVOR: That is a matter of concern.

(Cut to three weeks later)

"Breaking news from the Rikers Island Prison – two men tested COVID-19 positive of which one was a prisoner and the other a jailor," the voice of a reporter speaking on TV came from the Superintendent's office.

This caused a state of unrest in the prison.

The two men were admitted to the ICU but the treatment didn't seem to work. They were soon declared dead by the doctors of the COVID-19 unit. Their bodies were loaded in refrigerated trucks and sent off to Hart Island for burial.

The burial team in charge recorded the casualties:

Coffin 78C- Stuart Binge, Coffin 79C- Belle Troy, Coffin 80C- **Stephen Smith,** and Coffin 81C- **Trevor Laddy**.

Their coffins were laid next to each other. And they rest thus for eternity.

The corona virus makes no distinction. It affects all the same way, irrespective of their deeds, their thoughts and their perspectives on life. People, good and bad, are on the same boat in this war against COVID-19. What is man-made is of little significance when it comes to wars like this.

> Let the dead
> Bury the dead
>
> "Harper Lee"

The Affidavit

"**S**ir, *jaan haazir hai aapke liye*! (My four brothers and I will lay down our lives for you)."

Naresh never held back while declaring his admiration for Dr.Krishna Kumar aka KK. KK, who was a well known surgeon in Haripur town of Uttar Pradesh, had helped Naresh find his feet in medical practice. Naresh considered him his mentor and guru. He freely admitted that he owed much in his career to KK. Often Naresh would go a bit overboard while making grandiose loyalty affirmations towards Dr. KK.

"Do you know the story of Guru Govind Singhji and his *panj pyare*?" KK asked Naresh.

"Sir, forget the story, you should know that you can count on me for anything, anytime. If I hesitate for even a second to obey you, I will ride through the whole town on a donkey with a blackened face," said Naresh, hero worshiping KK as usual.

"Ha, ha, ha, that's fine, Naresh. But listen to the story first. It dates some 300 years back to 13

April 1699 in Anandpur Sahib. It was the occasion of Baisakhi, and *kirtan* was on. Suddenly the *dasham* (tenth) guru Govind Singhji stood up with an unsheathed sword in hand and called out to the crowd seeking human sacrifices for the sake of the faith. He asked whoever was ready to volunteer his life for the faith to come forward.

One brave man stepped up and offered his head. Guruji took him inside a tent. Outside people heard sounds of a sword slicing flesh. There was blood in the drain which flowed from his tent. Guruji came out of the tent with blood on his sword and asked if there was any other volunteer. Another brave man came forward and Guruji took him inside as well. The process was repeated five times. The assembly was stunned.

After the whole charade was over, Guruji came out with the five brave men now dressed in saffron and a turban. Guruji called them his 'panj pyaarey'- the beloved five. Guruji offered them a drink of sugared holy water from the Sutlej river in an iron bowl, stirred with a '*khanda*'- a double-edged sword. He said the five had been reborn as part of a new brotherhood, and gave them the surname 'Singh' (meaning lion). Thus, the martial khalsa was born to counter the constant oppression of the Mughal regime.

So, my dear Naresh, when the time comes, I will certainly remember your words," said KK, finishing his story. Though he said it ironically, even KK didn't know that such a time would soon come.

......

One Sunday, early in the morning at about 5 am, KK received a phone call.

On the other side was a member of KK's hospital staff.

"Sir, Rajesh is lying unconscious on the floor in the OT (Operation Theatre)," the man said.

"Try to wake him up. He may have drunk too much. I am coming," KK said. He soon left for the hospital. He lived in doctors' apartments on the hospital campus and it didn't take him long to reach the operation theatre.

The staff member who had called him, the night superintendent, and a few others accompanied him into the OT.

It turned out Rajesh had been dead for hours. His body was cold and stiff. He was lying next to the anesthesia trolley; the mask used to administer anesthesia was in his hand, close to his mouth.

KK noticed the anesthesia halothane jar in the trolley was empty. He remembered it had been almost full the previous day.

"There was no surgery last night. Why did Rajesh come to the OT at all?" KK asked.

"Sir two surgeries were scheduled early in the morning, so he stayed," someone answered.

"He was preparing surgical drums. He even said not to disturb him at night," someone else added.

"OT is a highly segregated area and surgery was planned for 7 am. How did you find him?" KK asked the staff member who had phoned him.

"Sir, he had asked me to alert him at 5 am. I couldn't find him on his couch in the staff room, so I came here looking for him. I found him here in OT. I immediately informed you and others as well. Sir, he was addicted to halothane (the anesthesia vapour)."

"But you never told me that earlier," said KK. He was both angry and sad about the loss of a young life. He knew halothane vapor was highly addictive, but he had never imagined that someone from his staff could become an addict.

"Okay, let us inform the police and his parents as well," he said, taking a deep breath.

....

Rajesh had lost his mother while still a child. His father, Suresh, worked in another city. Rajesh lived with his stepmother and four step-siblings. The family had faced another tragedy two years back when one of the stepsisters committed suicide. The family was poor, with bare survival income. KK knew this and used to help Rajesh financially wherever he could.

Police reached the hospital soon after being informed. Rajesh's family also arrived along with some of their neighbors. KK made arrangements to help Rajesh's father Suresh return to the town the same day. Police planned for postmortem, which could not be done on the family request. Dr. KK and others in the hospital advised the family to let the police do a postmortem, but Suresh remained unwilling. He gave the police a written statement that he would not engage in any legal proceedings related to the death later. Eventually the police gave in to Suresh's wishes.

Rajesh was cremated the very next day without a postmortem.

Two days after Rajesh's death, Suresh visited Dr. KK along with two relatives. KK thought they had come to settle any remaining formalities at the hospital. He got the shock of his life when they asked him to pay them Rs 500,000 or face the consequences.

"Suresh Ji, my sympathies are with you and your family. But you also need to understand that like other people here, I'm also only paid a salary. This sum is too large for me to give you. Still, Rajesh was part of our team and we will try to help your family in whatever way we can," he assured Suresh.

Though the hospital provided no help, KK and his staff started a voluntary fund and helped the family by collecting some money and handing it over.

But Suresh wasn't satisfied.

He saw an opportunity in the tragedy. Unable to extract the expected ransom from KK, he lodged an FIR against him and his staff claiming they had murdered his son.

Though the complaint was made three months after the death, the next day's headline in local newspapers read, "Famous surgeon of Haripur booked in murder case."

KK was disheartened and helpless.

"The truth shall prevail. Let the police investigate thoroughly," was his only statement to journalists.

The police started their probe. The investigating officer collected the required facts, details of the OT where the corpse was found, statements of the staff on duty, the doctors, and Rajesh's parents. All were asked to submit sworn affidavits.

The allegations and investigation took their toll on the working atmosphere of the hospital. Many rumors were in the air. It seemed as if everyone had his own theory of what had happened. Amidst all this, Suresh came to KK with a proposal to settle the case. Suresh said he would take back the case if KK was ready to pay Rs 200,000. KK refused.

One day soon after, KK was sitting with a friend, Sanjeev, when Naresh walked in. Sanjeev had been friends with KK for many years and knew Naresh too. Sanjeev pulled up a chair for Naresh.

"Sir, you are looking tense," said Naresh sitting down.

"Naresh, you know what has been happening," Sanjeev answered for KK.

"One can't relax unless the whole thing is over. There are so many things that come to mind. Police may even arrest KK for a crime which has not happened," Sanjeev continued. "It could occur even in your presence Naresh."

Sanjeev had touched Naresh's raw nerve. He was aware of Naresh's habit of boasting undying loyalty to KK.

"Why didn't you say anything earlier, sir? My brothers and I would lay down our lives for you," said Naresh, standing up excitedly.

Sanjeev looked at KK, both smiled.

"Oh yes-yes, I had forgotten my lion," KK said, smiling.

"Sir, you please relax. You need not to worry as long as I am here. I will be with you till my last breath," Naresh said.

"Naresh, all of us have to give affidavits to the police of the required facts," KK said.

"Okay, sir. Sanjeevji, please make an affidavit saying whatever has to be said to save sir and I'll sign it," said Naresh, before leaving.

KK and Sanjeev looked at each other.

"Sanjeev, this is the time to test our lion. Make an affidavit saying what I tell you to, and get Naresh's signature. You have to insist that he read it and then sign," KK instructed Sanjeev.

"Yes, got it. He does exactly the opposite of what, is insisted to do", Sanjeev smiled and went to a lawyer to prepare the affidavit.

....

A day later, KK, Naresh, and a few other friends were all seated at KK's house. Sanjeev entered the room waving a piece of paper, and carrying his briefcase.

"Everyone, I want to give you good news. But before that, I want all of you to applaud Naresh. It's all because of him," Sanjeev said.

Everyone cheered.

"Now tell us the good news, Sanjeev," asked KK.

"Well, now no one needs to worry about anything. Dr Naresh has taken care of everything. Isn't that true, Naresh," Sanjeev announced.

"Yes of course, I have signed the affidavit. No one can touch KK Sir as long as I am alive," said Naresh.

"Naresh did you read the affidavit before signing it," KK asked.

"Sir, whatever is written on it, I will own. Believe me, sir, I and my brothers ...."

"Wait, wait," KK stopped him. "Sanjeev, will you read it aloud for all of us?"

"Sure KK. It's Naresh's great sacrifice, everyone should know. I have submitted the original affidavit to the deputy superintendent of police, so I will read from the Xerox copy that I have brought," Sanjeev said.

Sanjeev opened the affidavit and started reading-

"I, Dr. Naresh, s/o Raj Singh R/O Buddha Garden, Haripur, state on oath that..."

Sanjeev looked around the room. Everyone was eager to know how Naresh had single handedly solved KK's problem, while none of them had been able to..

"Go ahead Sanjeev ji, why have you stopped," Naresh said proudly with a 56 inch chest.

Sanjeev read: "**On Midnight Of April 1, I Killed Rajesh, S/O Suresh Chand, In OT-2 Knowing Fully What I Was Doing ...**"

Naresh's jaw dropped. Small beads of sweat appeared on his forehead. He felt as if someone had sucked the air out of his lungs. He struggled to stand up. His legs trembled.

"Sanjeev Ji, what are you reading. This was not in the affidavit. You must be joking" said Naresh, taking several deep breaths.

"Naresh, I gave you the affidavit to read and told you only then to sign it. It was with you for more than 10 minutes. How could you have missed this?" Sanjeev said with a blank expression.

Naresh's face went pale.

"Let me complete now," Sanjeev said, and resumed reading

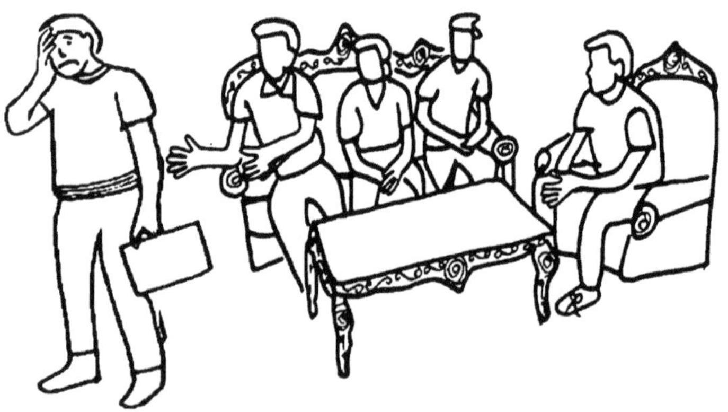

"My Motive For Killing Him Was That He Kept Repeatedly Challenging My Manhood, and No One Else was my Associate in this Cruel and Evil Act."

Suddenly Naresh jumped up and snatched the affidavit from Sanjeev's hands.

"You cheated me!!!"

He became hysterical and started crying.

"Ab kya hoga (what will happen now). I have not seen anything in life. I haven't even married. My life, my career are finished. I am dead now. I will call my brothers, my mother. They will take revenge," he began to yell, beating his chest. Unable to breathe, he fell down, started to roll on the floor and fainted.

When he opened his eyes, he saw both Sanjeev and KK's faces. Sanjeev and KK were sprinkling water on his face. They lifted him off the floor and put him on a bed. He was still trembling, and breathing fast. He kept murmuring, "Sanjeev Ji, you cheated me, Sanjeevji you cheated me."

Sanjeev now unlocked his briefcase. He took out the original affidavit, and placed it in Naresh's hand. "Take it back," he said.

KK smiled. "Naresh my lion, relax," he said. "Neither it is Baishakhi, and nor are we in Anandpur Shahib. Those were extraordinary men who had the capacity to sacrifice their all for a noble cause. I can't expect that from you. So, nobody will make you sacrifice your life or take your head. We didn't submit that affidavit to the authorities."

Everyone was smiling, except Naresh, who held the affidavit in his hand. He still couldn't believe what had happened in last 10 minutes.

At first he couldn't dare to read the last lines, but finally did.

EVERYTHING SAID ABOVE IS UNTRUE. THE DOCUMENT IS MADE FOR THE PURPOSE OF FIRST APRIL ONLY. GOD WILL HELP ME.

He looked around at everyone and then at his signature at the bottom of the document, which appeared to him like a snake with its fangs ready to strike him.

If a June night could talk, it would probably boast it invented romance.

"Bernard Williams"

When boasting ends, there dignity begins.

"Owen D Young"

A Soldier Born Again

"I want a baby," said the old lady groveling with folded hands...

"Everyone sitting here wants a baby.....Amma," said Dr. Vimlesh with a smile. "Just sit down and tell me about it."

Dr Vimlesh ran the only test tube center in Haripur. Counseling people this way was routine for her. Almost daily, there were young women coming to her for help to have a baby by any means. Sometimes it was their mothers who came. She would make them comfortable and first listen to their stories.

"Madam, I want a baby, the old woman repeated." "Okay, Amma. I got you. But babies are not gifted here, they are born here."

"Ji Madam, I know that."

"So call your daughter or daughter in law on whose behalf you have come."

"I am here for myself, Doctor Madam."

"Meaning?"

"Meaning, I want to get pregnant."

"At your age? Are you crazy, old lady?" Dr. Vimlesh looked her from head to toe.

"Yes, I want a baby and I am crazy for one."

"Pregnancy is not possible at your age. Don't you know that? How old are you?"

"Yes I am 60 years old doctor."

"So at this age why are you so crazy for a baby? At this age usually people have so many health ailments. Nature does not favor pregnancy at this age."

"Doctor Madam, the test tube baby process is also not natural. I want a baby from my womb at any cost. Do whatever you want and can."

She looked stubborn, Dr. Vimlesh noticed. But being an experienced doctor and fertility expert it was her duty to counsel her humanely. She made a last effort.

"Amma, if you go for pregnancy at this age, you will need the eggs or the ovum of a young woman. It may even risk your life."

"You can take the eggs from my niece."

The old lady was adamant. "And sperms, though you had not mentioned them, are available." She called her husband, 65 years old.

Dr Vimlesh was speechless. With no option, she decided to get started on the long, painful process. She carried out all the required medical evaluations of the old lady from ultrasound and hormone testing to endoscopic examination of her womb.

As it happened, the retrieved eggs from her distant niece and the sperms of her husband were both of good quality. With hormone therapy, her barren womb became fertile.

In her very first attempt, she conceived. The fertilized egg was transferred to her womb and started growing. People started calculating the days to her delivery. And the awaited day came soon.

.....

"Congratulation Santosh, you are blessed with a baby boy." With time Dr. Vimlesh had started calling the lady by her name.

Santosh smiled. She tried to say something but felt shooting pain in her abdomen. She had tears, but she smiled again. The baby had been delivered by a C-section operation, and the pain, however intense, did not matter. Motherhood carries the extreme happiness of becoming a creator and feeling much the way Lord Brahma must have felt when He populated the universe with life.

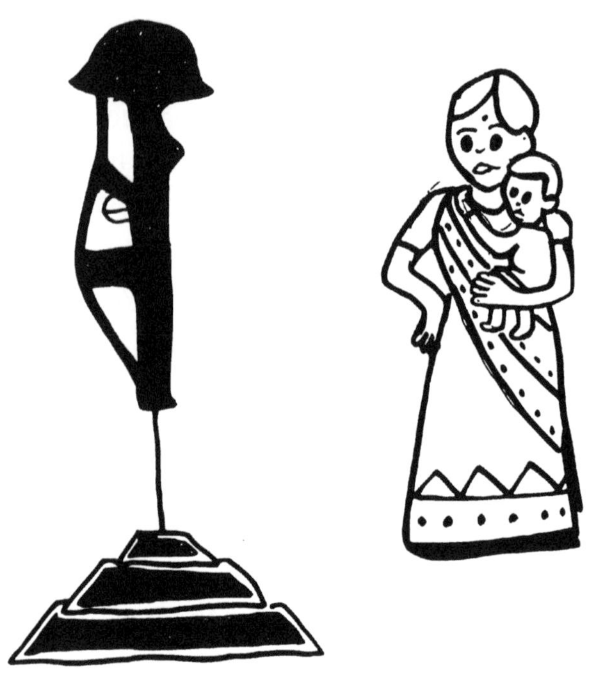

"Madam, some army man wants to see you." Mamta, a staff nurse and close associate of Dr. Vimlesh, informed her on the intercom.

"Sorry to disturb you madam, I just came to pay our respects on behalf of my unit. I am Commanding Officer (CO) of CRPF's Sukma unit, Chhattisgarh."

"You are most welcome sir, but I did not get you." Dr Vimlesh greeted him respectfully.

"Okay, I will make it easy for you. Actually, I'm conveying my sincere thanks to you personally for taking care of patient Santosh the mother of my young martyr, cadet Vijay Singh.

"Her son was a martyr when ... how?" Dr Vimlesh asked, her eyes wide open.

"He was my brave soldier and her only son. He was martyred in an ambush fighting Naxalites in 2014." He took a deep breath.

"My God, she never told me."

"Mothers of soldiers are like that. They never shed tears for their martyred sons. They keep their emotions inside. It only shows in their eyes. These are brave mothers of brave sons."

"That's true, brave mother of a brave son." Dr. Vimlesh nodded.

"One more thing," said the CRPF CO. "Vijay was martyred just before he was to get married. It happened the day before he was to go home. His last message to his fiancée was – Coming tomorrow with the wind. And to his mother he had said –...will sleep in your lap, Ma."

Dr Vimlesh covered her ears with both hands. Her eyes were wet. On both sides, the Naxalites and the security forces, sons of poor mothers were being sacrificed. It has been said that the Naxalite movement aims to bring justice to the oppressed classes, but she had never been convinced. The young CRPF boy martyred was also from a poor family. How could it be justified...... justice should be for all.

"May I meet the great mother and the newborn?" He requested, breaking her train of thought.

"Yes of course, sir." She personally escorted him to Santosh's room.

The Commanding Officer saluted the mother, congratulated her and blessed the baby.

Santosh was happy to see the officer. She wished him and briefly handed over the baby to him.

"It's your Vijay, sir, born again to serve you and the motherland," she said.

The baby was staring into the eyes of the commanding officer. Everyone else's eyes in the room were full of tears.

"Yes Vijay Singh .... my brave soldier...born again, the officer said."

> Let us all be brave enough to die the death of a martyr, but let no one lust for martyrdom.
>
> "Mahatma Gandhi"

Bhasmasur

Mahesh walked absentmindedly. He didn't have a destination in mind nor any urgency to go anywhere. He just wanted to get away. But he didn't know what he wanted to get away from. He didn't realize when he left the main road and started walking down a narrow trail. His trance was broken by a voice coming from a loudspeaker.

Coming to his senses, he looked around. He had come quite far from the main road. There wasn't much to see where he was standing. On one side of the trail, a peasant was sowing seeds on land that didn't look too fertile. On the other side was a vast stretch of land. In one corner was a structure which seemed half built. Bricks in the wall were bare and had been covered with mud instead of plaster. A tin shed tried to make up for the absence of a proper roof. A beggar sat outside the structure looking at Mahesh with hope in his eyes. He begged Mahesh for some money for food. Mahesh ignored him. "What good has helping anyone brought me," he thought. He saw there was a loudspeaker tied to a pole on top of the tin roof. Mahesh noticed that the voice coming from the loudspeaker had a strange calmness and an enchanting effect. The sound was deep and yet its texture was smooth. The speaker was probably inside the structure. Out of curiosity, Mahesh entered it.

It was an ashram. On a small stage in front was a person sitting cross legged and speaking into a mike. Mahesh wasn't able to guess his age. His hair was completely white, but his face had a glow, which is seen only in a person in his prime. He even had a small audience. As Mahesh listened, he noticed that people were addressing the speaker as Guruji.

Guruji was narrating the story of Bhasmasur and Lord Shiva.

"Bhasmasur was a great devotee of Shiva. He worshipped Shiva for years and performed great penances. Pleased with his devotion, Shiva said he was willing to grant him a boon. Bhasmasur cleverly asked for the power to turn anyone whose head he touched into ashes.

"'So be it,' said Shiva.

But such great power didn't go well with Bhasmasur. It corrupted him. He thought that with such power he could get anything he wanted. Blinded by his desire, he wanted Shiva's wife,

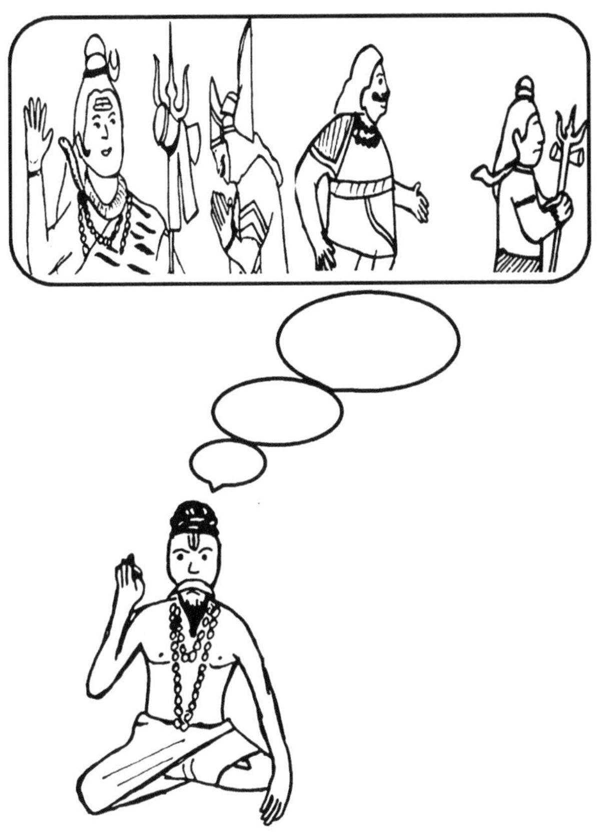

Goddess Parvati. "To get Parvati, I must first get Shiva out of my way," he thought. In his foolish pursuit, he attempted to touch Shiva and burn him. Realizing his evil intention, Shiva fled from him, while Bhasmasur kept pursuing him.

Shiva sought help from Lord Vishnu. Vishnu agreed to help and took the form of a beautiful woman, Mohini, and appeared in front of Bhasmasur. Attracted by Mohini's divine beauty,

Bhasmasur forgot about Parvati and Shiva and asked Mohini to marry him.

Lord Vishnu, in the form of Mohini, replied that "she would only marry a person who matched her dancing skills."

Bhasmasur accepted Mohini's challenge and said that "he could match all her dance moves."

Seeing that Bhasmasur had taken the bait, Mohini started dancing. Whatever dance moves she performed, Bhasmasur was able to match them. While dancing, Mohini struck a pose where she put her hand on top of her own head. Moving with the flow, Bhasmasur imitated her and touched his own head. He was immediately turned into ashes as per the boon he had received from Shiva.

"So, what do we learn from this story?" Guruji asked. He himself answered. "The moral of the story is that we shouldn't be distressed if we supported and empowered someone, and that person then uses the very tools and power we gave them to harm us. Don't think of your act of trusting someone as a mistake. Just keep doing your "Karma" and you will get its results. Don't worry about the people who forgot what you did for them, as their own karma will take care of them just as it did with Bhasmasur."

Guruji had finished the story. People started moving out after touching his feet and obtaining his blessings. After everyone left, Guruji noticed that one person was still sitting lost in thought. It was Mahesh.

Guruji went to him and gently touched his shoulder.

“Are you okay, son?” Guruji asked with love.

“I have created a Bhasmasur!!” said Mahesh, his eyes fixed on some unknown distant point.

“What?” Guruji was a bit confused

“Forgive me, Guruji. I didn’t realize the satsang is over. I should also go,” Mahesh said, realizing he was the only one left behind.

“That’s okay, son. You look worried. You said you have created a Bhasmasur. What is it about? Tell me, what has been worrying you?”

Mahesh wasn’t sure how to discuss his situation. He hesitated in narrating his problems to Guruji.

“You can tell me. Don’t worry. Even if I am not able to help you, at least I will share your pain,” Guruji said.

“It was my foolishness Guruji, he ditched me.” Mahesh took a deep breath. There were tears in his eyes.

“Here, have a glass of water. Have faith in God and have faith in yourself.”

Mahesh drank water, and collected his strength to speak.

"Guruji, his name is Rakesh. I brought him to my city from the village. He was doing menial jobs there despite being educated. His father had requested me to find him a job in the city. He wanted his son to do some work that would do justice to his education. Rakesh's father had gone through many difficulties to get him educated and was disappointed that he was not able to find a decent job. At his request, I arranged a clerical job for him in the city. Wherever I went, I presented him like my younger brother. He also worked hard and my faith in him grew with time. Soon he became my close associate and partner in almost all spheres of my life, including professionally, in all my ups and downs.

He was by my side at each step. I took him to clubs and introduced him to the city's elite. I trusted him so much that I even gave him the power of attorney for my business. If only I had known that by giving this power to him, I had put my neck in his hands.

Slowly my companies ran up debts despite doing good business. He took loans from the market and from banks using my goodwill, but did not pay them back. I had started many business projects in his name in good faith. He threw me out of them, even though majority of them were funded by me. He pushed me to the verge of becoming a defaulter to banks and the market."

Mahesh stopped for a while.

"Not only that guruji; whenever I tried to clear up things with him, he would defer the discussion on some pretext or other. Meanwhile I learnt that he had planned a coup to remove me from my own businesses. When I became a little strict in dealing with him, he left the business, taking away with him some of my key staff members, leaving me with all the liabilities he was responsible for. He threatened to ruin me. He had always been more vocal than me. He started defaming me all around. He was the mastermind and informer behind an income tax raid on me. He has been speaking of my wife, who cared for him like a son, in such language that I can't even repeat his words," he continued.

"Guruji, I did nothing wrong to him. It was I who raised him to this stature he acquired. And now he is trying to ruin me with the money and power I gave him. I don't know what to do. I have lost all my faith in humanity and my interest in life, in business and mankind. Sometimes I want to punish myself. It was my mistake and my bad decision. I feel like a beggar roaming the roads, losing my business and my hard-earned respect. Should I just give up? I don't know how I will be able to trust anyone again in life."

"Son, I understand how you are feeling," said Guruji. "But although you heard the Bhasmasur story you didn't understand it fully, or you probably misunderstood it. The story was not about how you should not trust people or how people will take advantage of you if you help them succeed. Lord Shiva is the supreme god. He knows about our past, present and future. You can fairly assume that he knew what was going to happen when he gave the boon to Bhasmasur. Still, he did so because that was the fruit of the penance and devotion of Bhasmasur. That was his good karma, and Shiva had to reward it.

Similarly, Bhasmasur's bad karma and wrong intention led to his fall. Don't you think that Shiva, being the ultimate destroyer in the universe, could have easily eliminated Bhasmasur? But he went to Vishnu because it had to be Bhasmasur's lust and arrogance that would cause his death.

So son, if the supreme God can trust a person knowing that he will turn into an enemy, how can you call yourself a fool for trusting someone? On the contrary, it makes you a courageous person."

Mahesh felt as if a weight had lifted from his chest. The darkness of his pessimism had been dissolved by the wise words of Guruji. He touched Guruji's feet and came out of the ashram. Before starting on his way back, he took out his wallet, picked out the biggest currency note in it and handed it to the beggar.

The peasant on the other side of the trail was still watering his land. The land didn't look so barren to Mahesh now.

> A friend is nothing but a known enemy.
>
> "Kurt Cobain"

Sundar And The Monkey Child

Throughout our lives we come across many relationships. There are a few we are born with while others we build in this journey of life. One of the most beautiful relationships is that between a child and its parents. But it would be our false pride if we thought that humans were the only ones to experience this incredible bond. On the contrary, it is one of the strongest instincts inherent in all animals and birds.

Unfortunately, in our arrogance of being the smartest species, we often turn a blind eye to this aspect of animal behavior, which can even teach us how to honor a relationship. But sometimes we come across instances which give us a whole new perspective, which teach us that certain emotions transcend the boundary of the species we belong to. I was a witness to one such incident.

"Sunder!!! I am starving, send my lunch to my room," I yelled even before entering the mess, and turned to go to my room without waiting for the answer.

But it wasn't exactly my fault that I was in such a rush. I had been on duty for 30 hours straight. During those 30 hours, I was the only house surgeon in Emergency and had been attending to emergency surgeries one after another. Most people sympathize with a person who is undergoing surgery, but not many people are aware of what the house surgeon in the emergency ward of a medical college undergoes. Had they known how that poor fellow carries the burden of responsibility of the whole department on his shoulders, they might shed a tear for him too.

When my shift ended, I was mentally and physically exhausted. I hadn't slept at all and the only food I had eaten was two chapatis which an intern had graciously offered. Now all I wanted was some food and a bed to crash on. Thankfully I found a colleague who gave me a lift to my hostel.

As soon as I reached my hostel I went to the mess and asked Sundar to send lunch to my room.

"Mess is closed sir, no lunch today." Sundar said with his head hanging low.

Sundar was our cook or "*Maharaj*". Nobody knew when or how he came to our hostel from Nepal. For all students, he was like an elder brother.

It wouldn't be right to say he didn't have a family as he considered all students his family – a very big, dynamic family which every year some new members joined and some old ones left to find their own place in the larger world outside.

Despite these regular changes in family membership, it was surprising how Sundar remembered each and every member and ex-member's face, even if a person was coming back to college after 10 or 12 years. Whenever an old student visited, Sundar's happiness knew no bounds. The kind of joy he felt was probably similar to a grandfather seeing his grandson after years. You would see tears in his eyes. In all those years, we had never seen Sundar refusing to serve a meal no matter what odd time we asked for it. In a hostel of doctors, such requests were quite regular due to our irregular schedules and nature of work. So, what had happened today?

"Has someone died, what the hell is going on?" I was almost yelling. I rarely shouted, but fatigue and hunger had made me bitter.

"Yes sir. Someone died."

It was like somebody threw cold water over a raging fire. All my anger evaporated in an instant.

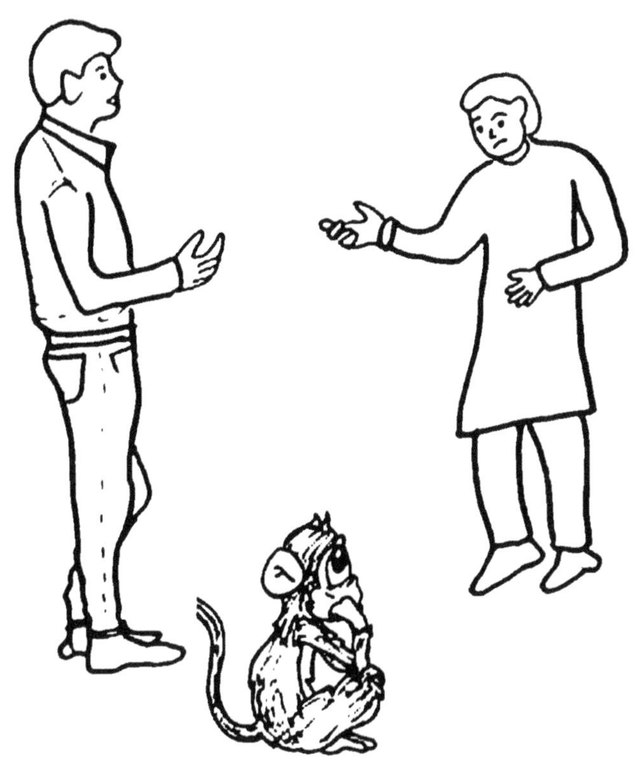

“What??” My bag dropped from my hand. I turned to face him.

“Who?” I asked

“A monkey!” He said in a trembling voice. His face had gone pale and his eyes were getting moist.

“A monkey! What monkey? No monkey resides here. You are confusing me, Sundar. Tell me exactly what happened.” I even forgot how tired I was.

"It was a female monkey. She died because of my mistake," Sundar started sobbing.

"Sir, come with me," he said.

"Where I wondered, but thought it would be best to just follow him.

I followed him inside our mess kitchen without uttering another word.

As he opened the mess door, my eyes met two glaring eyes which were like sparkling crystal. A cute infant monkey was staring at me with its big eyes.

I was not expecting this, to say the least.

"I thought you said the monkey died. Where have you got this from? Why are you keeping him?" I had a thousand questions for Sundar.

"The female monkey had this baby monkey with her. The mother monkey died because of my mistake. Now it's my responsibility to take care of him," Sundar said in a firm voice.

While I was trying to make some sense of what was happening, Sundar gave the baby monkey, which was tied to a window grill with a thin rope, some milk and bread. But the monkey didn't even look at the food. His eyes were searching for someone else.

"Sundar, I think you should release him. He belongs to the open," I advised him.

"No sir, now I am his guardian, his caretaker. I committed a sin today. Do you know what day of the week is today?" he asked.

"It is Tuesday, Hanumanji's day and look what has happened," he answered without waiting for me to reply.

"I pray to Lord Hanuman daily and I killed a monkey, a descendent of Lord Hanuman on a Tuesday," he started weeping.

I let him cry. Hanuman is the monkey God and the killing of a monkey is unpardonable for his followers. Tuesday is also known to be the day of Lord Hanuman and this poor devotee had committed this sin. It must be quite a painful condition for him.

"This monkey child came with his mother today morning. He was in her arms. She came and sat outside this window, so I gave her a few bananas and bread. But after that, she picked one of my shirts that I had hung outside to dry. I ran behind her to get it back, but she jumped and climbed over the rooftop there.

He pointed to a TV antenna, which coincidently I had put up on the roof for my black and white TV.

"When I came to the roof, she was sitting on the TV antenna," Sundar continued. "By this time I had gotten irritated and thought that she would tear my shirt, so I threw my wooden stick at her."

"Did that hit her?" I asked

"No, the stick didn't reach anywhere near her, but she jumped off the antenna. She dropped my shirt and jumped onto the top edge of the wall. But she could not maintain her balance on the narrow wall which broke away and she fell about forty feet. I ran downstairs immediately. But by the time I reached she was already dead.

"You know sir, she could have survived if she had tried to land on her hands or feet, but she used her arms to hold the child up and save him from the impact. She saved her child from even a minor injury, but it cost the poor creature her life." There was reverence in Sundar's voice for the monkey.

"Sundar, all mothers are like that." I patted him on the shoulder.

"Have you performed her last rites?" I asked.

"Yes sir, I cremated her with all the rites and prayed for her soul. And I have adopted her child. But sir, I will not forgive myself. I don't know why I had to throw that stick at her. It all happened because of this damn shirt!" He suddenly jumped and threw the shirt, which was lying in a corner, in the mud oven he used for making chapatis. The room was filled with the smell of burning polyester.

"Sundar, it was accidental. You did the right thing by adopting her child. Many things are pre-decided. You didn't do it on purpose so don't feel guilty. I know you will take good care of her child." I tried to console him.

....

It was the third day after the incident. And it felt as if not only Sundar, but the whole hostel had adopted the baby monkey. Whoever went to the kitchen would give a part of his meal to the baby. The monkey had also become somewhat familiar with the setting. He wasn't anxious anymore in the presence of people, and when I offered him a buttered toast, he happily took it from my hand.

I came to my room and switched on the TV. But all that came on the screen was static. I asked my friend Anil to go and set the antenna in the right direction. Anil lazily got up from his chair and went out giving me a nasty look. He came back at twice the speed he had gone.

"There is a giant monkey sitting near our antenna," he said, breathing heavily.

I went back with him to the roof. Anil was right. It was probably the biggest monkey I had ever seen, and it was still there. We dared not touch the antenna.

“We can watch the news tomorrow or just read the newspaper,” we said to each other and came back.

After a few hours, in the evening, we again went to check the antenna. To our surprise, the giant monkey was still sitting there. Seeing us coming to the roof, he quietly came down from the antenna and sat on top of the broken wall from which the female monkey had slipped three days back.

For some time, we just stood there observing the monkey. But it was like he wasn’t bothered by our presence. We also didn’t have any intention of bothering him. So, we gathered all our courage to reach the antenna and corrected its direction. The monkey completely ignored us and sat there without moving. We came back to our room.

Later, our watchman told us that the monkey had been there since the morning and had been repeating a routine. He would sit on the TV antenna, then move to the broken border wall, then climb down to the spot where the mother monkey fell. “Initially, people were afraid of him, but he wasn’t concerned with us,” the watchman said. “We have tried to give him fruits, but he didn’t want them. He has been sitting there all day without eating or drinking."

……

Next morning, I went to the kitchen with some biscuits for the baby monkey. I whistled out to him, searching for those sparkly big eyes.

"Sir, he won't come." It was Sundar's voice.

"Why?"

"He has gone with his father." Sundar showed me the piece of rope that had been chewed to cut it.

"In the night a giant male monkey came, cut the rope with his teeth and took away the baby in his lap. Sir, the child was looking into my eyes till they disappeared," Sundar said, recalling the episode.

"You let him take away the baby? I know you had grown quite attached to it," I asked him.

"That's true, sir. But I took away the child's mother by mistake. I couldn't keep him away from his father too."

"And who knows, the child might return to visit me like some of you people do," Sundar said with a smile while handing me tea.

I dipped one of the biscuits I had brought for the baby monkey in the tea and ate it. I drank the tea, slurping loudly. I was repeating a childish act I used to do deliberately to attract my mother's attention.

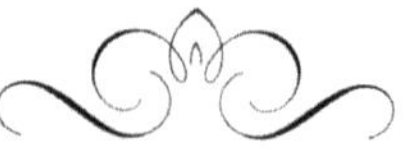

> Perhaps there is a soul hidden in everything and it can always speak, without even making a sound,to another soul.
>
> "Frances Hodgson Burnett"

Bicycle Thief

"Sir, may I have some milk," a kurta-pajama clad man asked Govind.

Govind was well known for his kind and helpful nature. Since the declaration of lockdown in India by the prime minister on 24th March 2020, following the corona virus pandemic, he had become very busy.

"Corona is a danger to all of mankind, and we have to come together to fight it," he had heard the PM say. He resolved to honor the PM's words. Unfortunately, his wife Madhu was not much impressed by his commitment.

"My parents made a big mistake when they married me with you," she muttered under her breath.

"Sethji, have you given a thought to saving something for your own children, or is that too much to ask for," she commented, pointing to their two daughters. It was only his wife who called Govind "Sethji" for being too generous to everyone while choosing a simple lifestyle for his own family.

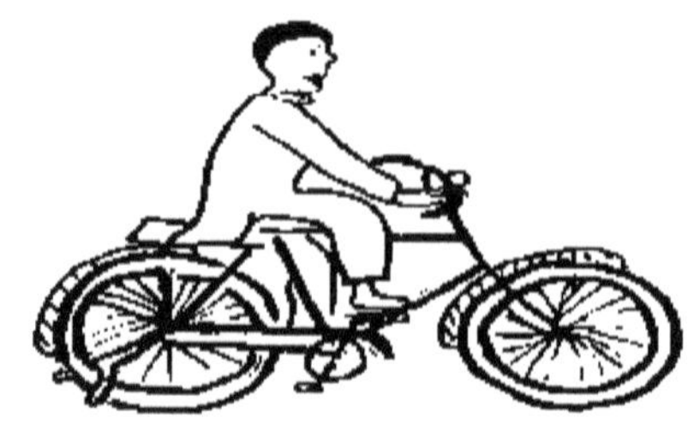

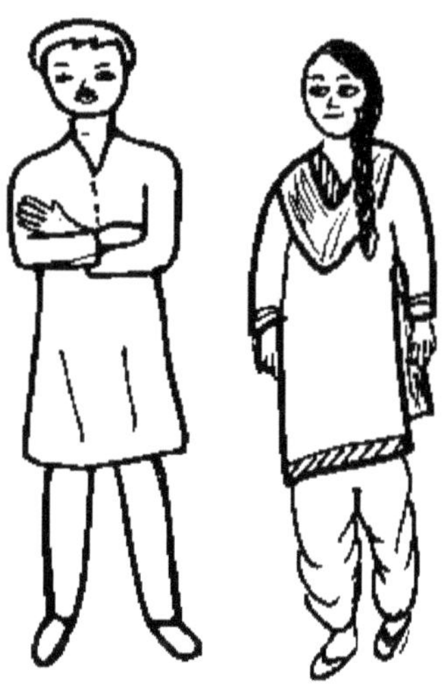

Govind had a small dairy on the city's outskirts. Behind his dairy, he had constructed a small home where he lived with his family. He had a beautiful Atlas bicycle which he had received as a marriage gift from his in-laws. He cared for it more than he did for himself. Every day after making his rounds of the market on it, he would clean it. Never once had he been negligent in taking care of it. Checking the air in its tyres, oiling the chain, putting grease in the brakes, was part of his routine. Even his daughters were fond of his cycle. When Govind took them to school on the bicycle, it was nothing less than a joyride at a fair for the girls.

His wife was even more possessive of the cycle than the other family members. Indian women are known to have a special affinity for the gifts they get from their parents.

Once, when Govind was returning from the city, his bicycle hit a pothole. He lost his balance and fell. An associate helped him get back home. As Govind's wife came out to open the gate for him she glanced at the cycle's handle, which had got crooked because of the accident.

"How can you be so careless with the bicycle that I had brought in the marriage," she hissed. She did a thorough inspection of the cycle, and only after being satisfied that the damage was not serious, went back inside. It was only a few moments later that she remembered Govind and came out with a glass of water, and asked, "Are you okay?"

"Yes, nothing serious," he smiled. He knew that she loved him with all her heart. She had been the one who had stood firmly with him in all the ups and downs of life. She was bitter with her tongue but sweet in her deeds. Govind always gave her credit for being more practical than him. Sometimes he would also get an earful from her, whenever someone took advantage of him, because he always put others needs before their own.

“Stop being so naïve. Not everyone in this world is as good as you think he or she is. People will make a fool of you if you aren’t careful,” she had advised him many times. “That’s why I married you dear, to balance my excesses,” Govind would say laughing.

“When you are on your best behavior, all gentle and nice, you become a devi, a Goddess,” Govind once said to her. “Let me remain a common woman. The Goddess will be angry with me if you raise me to her level, my Sethji,” she smiled and answered.

“Sir, my child is hungry, may I have some milk,” the man repeated.

Govind looked at him. “Okay. How much do you want?”

“Sir half a liter will be sufficient.”

“How old is your child?”

“He will be 10 year next month.”

“You seem to be from the east? Your accent suggests it.”

“You are right, sir. We are from Madhubani, Bihar.”

“How far it is from here?”

"It is about 1,200 km."

"My goodness! How are you planning to travel the distance?"

"We started on this bicycle from Ambala, which is almost 250 km from here. But before we reached here, the bicycle's chain broke. I was already struggling with the brakes. It's quite old and I don't know how far it will be able to carry us. But still, it's all I have. So, I have been dragging it now for almost 10 kms in the hope of finding a cycle mechanic, but haven't had any luck till now."

"It will be difficult to find a mechanic now. Everything is closed in the lockdown, bhaiya. How many family members do you have?"

"It's just me, my wife and a son. I left my wife and child in a shed nearby and came out here in search of food."

"Okay, you sit down and take some rest. Let me get the milk," said Govind, offering him a glass of water.

Govind went inside and returned with milk in a bottle, and some food in a packet. He asked his wife to make tea and also give the man something to eat.

"Here are some snacks for your journey, and some food for your wife and son," Govind said. Soon after, Madhu brought the tea.

“No, no sir. This is too much. I can’t take this. I don’t have much to give you in return,” the man said with folded hands.

“Bhaiya, I don’t want anything in return. It’s God’s will that He brought you to my doorstep, and we happen to have some extra food, as an expected guest didn’t turn up.” Govind lied. He understood the man had dignity and wouldn’t accept charity from him. He just hoped that he wouldn’t catch out his lie and ask how he had expected a guest despite the lockdown.

The man was overwhelmed by Govind’s hospitality and generosity. He took the food packet with great courtesy. Govind handed him tea.

“Destiny keeps testing these poor people. These innocent, hardworking people who have become helpless in the very cities they were helping to build. When they came, leaving behind their homes and families, they were poor, but they had dreams. Now disowned by everyone, they have lost their dreams too,” he thought. “All they wanted was an opportunity to work and earn their livelihood. They would have even gone to the moon if told there was work there. How distraught can it make a person when he doesn’t have hope for a better tomorrow? It’s happening not to one, but to thousands of people who are lining up like ants on the road, trying to get back home. If only I could have done something for them."

"There are not many people like you, sir, who would help a stranger. I don't want to trouble you anymore, but there is just one thing more I wanted to ask you if you don't mind," the man said hesitatingly as he sipped the tea.

"Yes, yes. Tell me. How can I help?" Govind said eagerly

"I noticed that you have a bicycle as well. Do you happen to have any spare chain I could use?"

"Actually, I don't have a spare chain as I don't use this cycle," Govind lied again.

"It's not even mine. Someone forgot it here a few years back, and since then I have just been taking care of it and waiting for the owner to return and claim it. It's just an extra chore for me daily." Govind finished his tea, collected the cups and went inside.

"I hope he got the cue," he said to himself.

When Govind came outside after a few minutes there was no sign of the man.

"Smart man," thought Govind. Just as Govind was appreciating the man's cleverness, Madhu came out.

"Where is my bicycle?" his wife cried.

"What! Oh, yes, it's missing. Where has it gone? It was here when I went inside," said Govind, acting surprised.

"You are always so careless; I know you wanted to get rid of my bicycle and of me too. I will not eat or drink anything until you find my bicycle," said Madhu. She went inside crying.

Govind stood there perplexed, wondering what to do next. He hadn't thought about how he would handle Madhu if the bicycle went missing. As he stood there, Madhu came out again. She was too restless to stay in the house.

"Will you just stand here all day, or do something? Go to the police station at least and file a report. And what's that near your foot?" she said, pointing to a piece of paper that had been carefully tucked under a stone.

Govind picked up the paper and started reading it. "Show me what it is." Madhu snatched the paper from his hand.

"My name is Abdul," she read. "I reside in Rafeek Nagar, Madhubani, Bihar. My son is physically challenged due to polio. He has walked his maximum physical limit. Now he is unable to even stand. I have no option to take him further except by stealing your bicycle. Please forgive me for the first theft of my life."

Madhu gasped for air before reading further.

"I will certainly come back after dropping my family at home to pay your debt. I am leaving behind my old bicycle at your place if it is of any use to you. Again, apologies for causing you trouble. I will keep you and your family in my prayers."

"Well, he confessed his crime. He has even given his address in the letter. This will be good proof for the police. Give the letter to me, and I will go to the police station," Govind said, testing her.

"Don't you dare to go to the police! Just take his old bicycle and get it repaired. I will pray to Lord Hanuman for their safe journey. My bicycle is being used for a good cause. You anyway didn't take good care of it. I will be happy with this old one." She went inside, to the idol of Lord Hanuman, and prayed for the family's safe journey.

Govind remained outside smiling at his good fortune to have got such an amazing wife who was praying for the thief who had stolen her prized bicycle.

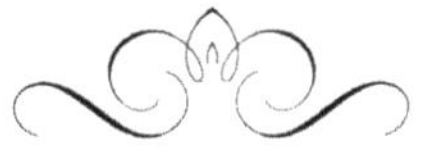

> Having a soft heart in a cruel world is courage, not weakness.
>
> "Katherine Henson"

THE ETERNAL BOND

Dr. Shruti hurried through her lunch in the hospital canteen. She worked at AIIMS, Bhubaneshwar, in the department of Medical Oncology. Being a doctor, and working with cancer patients, in particular, calls for total devotion and dedication. Dr. Shruti had these attributes.

But sometimes it was frustrating to find that while she cared for many, there was no one to care for her. Her husband, Rajiv, worked in a multinational company, and since the Covid-19 pandemic lockdown had begun, he was allowed to work from home, a luxury she as a doctor could not expect. But even then compelled to cook she never complained – and his phone calls kept disturbing her at work. It irritated her greatly.

"Why doesn't he understand that he is the one who gets to work from home, while I have so much to take care of at the hospital," she thought. "He can't keep calling me every two hours to 'just talk' to him. What a childish behavior!"

Finishing her lunch, she went to the tea vending machine, which had a clear view of the hospital's main gate, kept closed since the lockdown began, admitting only select arrivals. As she was pouring herself a cup, she couldn't help but notice an altercation at the gate. She walked carefully with the tea in her hand to where the hospital's security guard Pramod was arguing with an elderly stranger.

"You can't come in. Stop, I said STOP where you are!" exclaimed Pramod. The elderly man had been trying to push open the gate.

"Please let us in, it is an emergency," said the elderly man. "My wife needs help."

"I can't let you in. These are the orders and I can't make any exceptions. Since the lockdown all OPDs (Out Patient Departments) are closed," said Pramod. "Come back when the lockdown is over."

"...Please Sir, have mercy and let us in," begged the elderly man.

"Baba, don't make it harder for me than it already is," said Pramod. "Just leave."

"Bu..u..but sir, please at least listen to me first," the elderly man said, bowing desperately before Pramod.

Pramod nodded wearily, realizing the man would not leave otherwise, just as Dr. Shruti came close.

"Sir my name is Dashrath and this is my wife Savitri," said the elderly man, gesturing towards the frail, old woman with sunken eyes who stood next to him. "She has cancer. We have been coming here for her treatment for the last six months. Her appointment was actually a few days back, but we couldn't make it because of the lockdown. For the last two days, she has been in immense pain and weakness. Whatever medicines doctors had given were not providing any relief." He stopped to take a breath.

"We live about 140 kms away from here in a small village," he continued. "The only medical advice I could get in the village was from a compounder who stays near our house, who had worked for some years in a hospital. He told me her treatment must continue, that she needs chemotherapy and blood transfusion immediately.

"Sir, I work as a mason in the village. I neither have any conveyance nor money for an ambulance to bring her here. There is no public transport available because of the lockdown. But I couldn't see my Savitri in the condition she was in."

Before Dasharath could say any more, he stumbled. Pramod stopped him from falling, and gave him some water.

"I tried to get help from our village locals too, but they were as helpless as we were. I somehow got her to the highway near our village hoping some passing vehicle would give us a lift, but nobody would stop for a stranger, especially in these corona virus times. Finally, I picked up my rusty old bicycle and asked Savitri to sit on the carrier behind. She had become so frail due to the disease that she couldn't balance herself on to seat. So I tied her to my back and start pedaling"

"But you said you live 140 km from here," Dr. Shruti couldn't help interrupting.

"Yes, Doctor Madam." Dashrath realized that she was a doctor from the white coat and stethoscope she was wearing.

"So, you pedaled all the way here with your wife tied to your back!!" Shruti was staggered by the enormity of his achievement. "Yes, Doctor Madam. It's unfortunate to be poor in this world. But it's worse to be poor and ill because then there is no hope. I couldn't bear to see my wife in pain. I just couldn't...." Dashrath started sobbing.

At this point, his wife Savitri touched his shoulder. She tried to smile, despite the pain she was in.

Dr. Shruti couldn't hold back her tears either. Being a doctor, she had witnessed many tragedies at work. She had seen death from up close. It was the nature of her job. But what she was witnessing now was not tragic. It was the undying spirit of human nature, and of love.

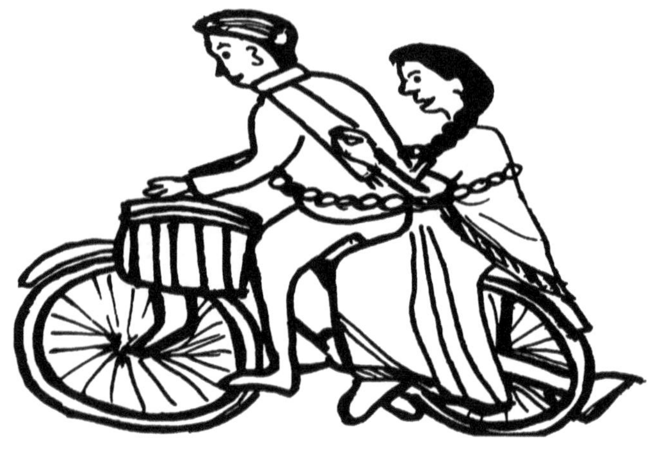

"Pramod, it's okay. Let them in," said Shruti firmly. Pramod opened the gate.

"Don't worry Dashrathji, nothing will happen to your Savitri. We'll take care of her & provide her treatment," said Dr. Shruti, as she took the bunch of old prescriptions Dashrath had been holding and rapidly went through them. Pramod assisted in getting a stretcher for Savitri, and helpers to carry her into the hospital.

"Our patient is 60 years old, female. She has liver cancer and looks severely anemic. Arrange four units of blood for transfusion and stabilize her vitals before preparing for chemotherapy," Dr. Shruti instructed her colleagues.

After a while, as her colleagues started the preparations she suggested, Dr. Shruti returned outside and called the security guard.

"Pramod, take that cycle the old man had used and see that it's parked somewhere safe. He had to pedal all the way here, but we won't let him go back the same way. I have talked to the senior doctors and the superintendent. At the time of discharge, we will ensure that there is an ambulance to take her and her husband home."

As Dr. Shruti walked back inside, she saw Dashrath sitting by his wife's side.

Dr. Shruti stopped. She remembered she had to call home. Savitri is fortunate to have such a caring husband, she said herself, having the utmost respect for Dashrath in her eyes.

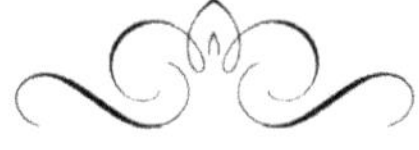

> One is loved because one is loved. No reason is needed for loving.
>
> "Paulo coelho"

The Bluff Master

“Isn't that Seema, boss?" Naresh asked Kumar. Even five year after he last saw her, he recognized Seema from a distance. After all, his best memories of college were linked to Seema. They had been close for the last three years of college. Unfortunately for Naresh, the relationship didn't go as he had hoped.

On the last day of college, inspired by too many Bollywood movies, Naresh had gone down on one knee and proposed Seema in front of the whole class. Seema wasn’t prepared for this bouncer. She was staggered but got her nerves together quickly and smashed that proposal right out of the boundary. Indian cricketers smash a spin bowler with more mercy. But Seema wasn’t one to mince her words.

"I don't know what goes on inside that head of yours, Naresh. I never gave any indication that I wanted to get married to you. College was different, but one has to be practical in life. I expect a lot from my life partner, and you can't fulfill those expectations!" She had said in front of everyone and left the room.

Naresh came from a lower middle class family and those words pierced his self-respect. He had zoned out and remained in that pose for a while even after Seema had gone. Finally, he stood up, but everything about him changed from that day. He became a person who valued outward appearance above everything else. He became a firm believer in the idea of "fake it if you can't make it".

And after five years, he now had a chance to show Seema what an opportunity she had missed by not marrying him. He wouldn’t miss it at any cost.

Naresh asked Prem Boss – as he called him – to stop the car they were travelling in just in front of Seema. Prem Boss was Naresh’s senior in the hospital they both worked at. Along with another colleague, Kumar, who had also been to college with Naresh but was also some years his senior, they were attending a conference in Meerut. Prem had bought a new Audi Q-7 and was itching to take it for a long drive. He found the excuse for it when he learnt of the conference.

"Come on Naresh, leave it. It's been a long time since that incident. She is married now and so are you. What's the point of this?" Kumar knew

Seema and Naresh's history and advised him not to do anything stupid.

"No, no boss. I just want to see how she is doing. I won't take that long. But please stop the car in front of her," Naresh pleaded to Prem.

"Okay, as you wish." Prem succumbed to his pleading.

"Thank you, thank you, boss," said Naresh, putting on his Rayban goggles.

As asked to, Prem stopped the car close to Seema. She was startled by the loud screeching of the brakes.

Naresh got out of the car, striking an attitude like a movie star.

"How are you, Seema?" said Naresh, taking off his Raybans. Their purpose had been fulfilled.

Seema, who was still in a bit of a shock from the car stopping so close to her and doubly surprised by seeing Naresh in front of her, went blank for a few seconds.

"I am good, Naresh. How have you been?" she finally replied, realizing she had been staring at Naresh for a while.

"Oh, I am very good. I am sorry you got startled by the car. I bought it last week. The driver is still getting used to it."

Seema was amazed, and so were Prem and Kumar. When had Naresh bought the Audi, and when had he employed Prem as his chauffeur?

Seema was also perplexed. Was this the same Naresh who had hardly a scooter while in college? How did he become so successful?

"By the way, I like your car too. Vintage!" Naresh chuckled, pointing to the Maruti 800 he had seen Seema stepping out of.

“Ha ha.... actually, my other car has gone for servicing, so I had to bring this,” Seema said, feeling a little uneasy.

“I need to go to the registration desk. I will see you later,” Seema said, and hurriedly left without waiting for a reply from Naresh.

“Yes, you can go anywhere you want. I have conveyed what I wanted to,” Naresh said to himself and went back to Kumar and Prem.

“So now I am your driver?” Prem said to Naresh.

“Sir, the way you supported me today, I will be your driver for life,” said Naresh. He laughed and touched Prem’s feet.

Bluffing was a regular habit with Naresh. Kumar and Prem knew it well. But today they had saved his dignity. Naresh had finally had his day, for which he had waited for years.

"That was okay for today, Naresh, but you need to be careful before saying anything to anyone. You might get in trouble someday," Prem advised before entering the conference hall.

....

It was about a month after this incident that Naresh met Kumar one day at the hospital where they worked, looking very pleased with himself.. They both lived in a town close to Delhi.

"Well, someone is having a good day," Kumar said to Naresh.

"Yes sir, it is a good day. Good day to teach people a lesson in respect and obedience," Naresh said proudly.

“Why? Who needed a lesson in respect and obedience?” Kumar was confused.

“A rickshaw wallah.”

"A rickshaw wallah?? What can a rickshaw wallah do to disrespect or disobey you?” Kumar wasn't smiling anymore. Though Naresh considered him a mentor, Kumar knew that sometimes Naresh's actions were beyond logic and sense.

“I hired him to bring me to the hospital.”

“So?”

“But then he picked one more passenger on the way and asked me to shift and make room for him. Can you believe it?”

“So?” Kumar was not able to comprehend what the rickshaw wallah had done wrong.

"How could he do that? I had hired him; he should have honored that agreement and carried me alone. He dared to make some stranger sit next to me." Simply recalling the incident was making Naresh hyper.

Kumar got it now. By asking Naresh to share his rickshaw seat, the poor rickshaw wallah had unknowingly pricked Naresh's sensitive ego.

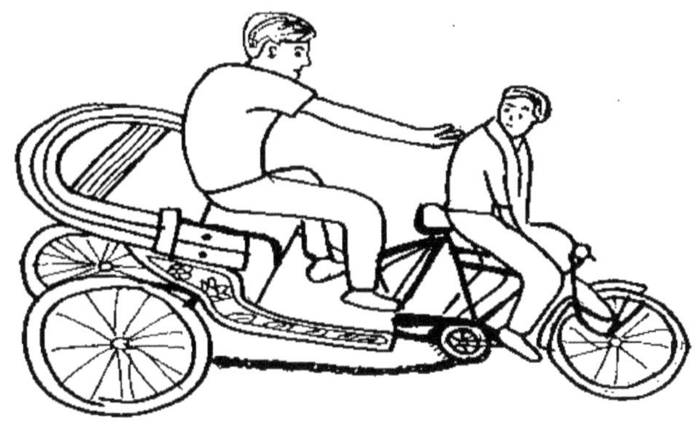

“But Naresh, how would it have harmed you? The poor guy was just trying to earn some extra fare from the other passenger in a single trip. If he didn’t have an issue with pulling double the weight, why would you deny him the opportunity?”

Naresh had not expected Kumar to take this contrary view. "But sir, I hired him first. If he wanted to take two passengers on the same trip, he should have told me. I wouldn't have hired him in the first place. I can't sit next to any odd person. Who knows if he is a thief or has some disease," said Naresh justifying his action.

"Naresh, he asked you to share the rickshaw seat, not to invite him to your home. The other passenger was also human, we all are equal." Kumar tried to put some sense into Naresh.

"Anyway, then what did you do," Kumar asked.

"I refused to move," Naresh said in a pompous voice.

“Then?”

“He asked me to step down from the rickshaw. He said he wouldn’t take me further. I warned him not to mess with me. I told him that if I wanted, I could ruin his life. But sir, he was a bull-headed person.

“He said he was a graduate, and yet driving a rickshaw. His life was already ruined. How could I ruin it further?”

Kumar realized that Naresh had met his match.

"That fellow was not ready to move. When I told him that I would call the police, he took me instead to the police station," Naresh continued.

“What happened then?” Kumar asked.

“Sir, it was an awkward situation for me. When I told the police officer about the incident, even he asked why I was making a ruckus over such a small matter. But then I gave him Rs 200 and told him to teach the rickshaw wallah a lesson. He gave the fellow two hard slaps. The rickshaw wallah will remember who he messed with,” Naresh said triumphantly.

“Then how did you come here?” Kumar was angry with Naresh by now, but tried not to show it.

"The same fellow dropped me here in his rickshaw. He had to be taught a lesson, taught to respect my dignity. I warned him that to work in our city he needed to learn manners. He should know who he is speaking to. We are the kings of this city," Naresh said.

"You lost my respect when you told me about getting him thrashed by bribing the police," Kumar thought. He took a deep breath. He felt this time Naresh had gone too far. He was the one who needed a lesson in respect.

“Okay Naresh, this rickshaw wallah, who is also a graduate, seems to have some self-respect. What was his name?”

“I did not ask, sir.”

"That's fine. Forget about it. You take care," Kumar said, and went into the operation theatre. He called a friend who was superintendent of a Government Hospital and gave him some instructions.

……

Two days later, the state chief minister was set to visit the city. Grand preparations for the visit were on at all levels. The whole administration was on its toes. Public servants were finally involved in public service. They were making every effort to ensure the chief minister, during his visit, would appreciate their work.

Just before the visit, Naresh came to Kumar, looking very worried.

"Sir I am in trouble."

"Trouble? What happened?"

"Sir, Kalwa has filed an FIR against me."

"Kalwa? Who is Kalwa?"

"Sir, the rickshaw wallah! The one I got beaten up by the police."

"Oh yes. Now I remember. You told me about him."

"Yes, sir."

"I had told you he seemed to be a man with self-respect. Anyway, what you did was wrong."

"Sir, forget wrong or right for now. First, help me."

"Hmmm... but how do you know he has filed an FIR?"

"Sir, I got a call from a police inspector. He told me that a person named Kalwa had filed an FIR against me. And that too under IPC section 307 - attempt to murder. I never touched him, sir. It was the policeman who did, and he too only slapped him."

"Yes, but you paid the policeman to beat him."

Sir, again you are going into irrelevant detail. More important is the fact that the FIR includes his medical report, which says he had a broken nose and bruises all over his body. How is it possible? He got only two slaps."

"Yeah. That's true. How could it happen?"

"Yes, that's the point. I told the Inspector who phoned me that the medical report must be false. But then he told me that it was prepared at the Government Hospital, so its authenticity can't be questioned."

"Did you speak to the doctor who prepared the report?"

"Yes, sir It was Dr. Lal. I called him and told him that I am a doctor too. I told him all that had happened that day. And though he was sympathetic, he said he couldn't do much. He told me that sometimes, to strengthen such cases, people do inflict injuries on themselves. Maybe that's what happened.

“Also, this Kalwa has support of the entire rickshaw wallahs’ union. Dr. Lal said they came to the hospital in a big group. The inspector was also saying that the union leaders were pressuring him to arrest me, or they would protest before the Chief Minister during his visit. Sir, even if I somehow escape arrest, they will protest in front of the CM. If it comes to the CM's notice, my license would surely be cancelled. And if I get arrested, my whole reputation and career will go down the drain. I am finished whatever happens. I don't know what to do." Naresh broke down.

"It’s a difficult situation, Naresh. Let me think about what we can do."

“Sir, save me. Save my career, my respect. My life will be ruined if I get arrested and jailed. ”, he cried.

“Naresh, do calm down. I had warned you earlier too that your excessive ego would take you down one day. Now see what has happened.”

Two warm teardrops fell from Naresh's eyes.

“Okay, let’s talk to Dr. Lal first,” said Kumar. “I know him personally. Maybe he can help us to find Kalwa’s address and then we can try to assuage Kalwa and get him to withdraw his FIR.” He dialed Dr. Lal’s number from his mobile and went out of the room to speak to him. He soon returned.

"Luckily, Dr. Lal has Kalwa's address in the hospital records," he said. "He is sending it to me. But he can do only so much. After that it is up to us to pacify Kalwa."

"Sir, the only person who can do it is you. I will do anything, sir; please see to it that Kalwa takes the complaint back." Naresh finally saw a ray of hope.

"Okay, Naresh. If I have to plead with a rickshaw wallah for your sake, so be it," Kumar sighed.

..

The Chief Minister visited and left after making many promises for the city's development. People were happy with the hopes of development he raised. The city's administration was happy as the visit had passed off smoothly. But one person's happiness outmatched everyone else's. Naresh had been saved from imminent arrest. To add to his joy, Kalwa had agreed to take back the complaint after Kumar visited him and apologized on Naresh's behalf. Initially Kalwa had been adamant on punishing Naresh, Kumar told him, but Kumar's humility had won him over.

To celebrate his escape and express his gratitude, Naresh promised Kumar a dinner at a five-star hotel in Delhi.

Dr. Kumar, Dr. Prem, and Dr. Lal were sitting in a restaurant at Hotel Taj Mansingh in Delhi waiting for Naresh.

"Full marks for your creativity, Kumar. You should be a scriptwriter for films," said Prem laughing.

Kumar and Dr. Lal smiled.

"It's nothing," said Kumar. "Naresh had unknowingly provided me with all the ingredients for the story. Add to this Dr. Lal's talent for changing his voice. I wanted to cure Naresh of his outsized ego and habit of bragging. You have the perfect story of Kalwa and his revenge!"

"Amazing. So, you never went to Kalwa's home?" said Prem.

"I didn't know who that poor rickshaw wallah was," said Kumar. "But I wanted Naresh to realize his mistake. So, I concocted the story of Kalwa and that he wanted to file an FIR. When there was no Kalwa, how would I have found his house? I just wanted to punish Naresh for the way he behaved with that poor rickshaw wallah. All we needed to do was make Dr. Lal change his voice and call him, pretending to be a police inspector.

"..And I added the story of rickshaw union to make the scenario more realistic," Dr. Lal said smiling.

"And that inspector?"

"Again, that was me calling from a different number, in an altered voice. When there is a call from the police station people often forget their own names. Fear of police!" said Dr. Lal. They all laughed.

They laughed till their stomachs began to hurt. Naresh reached a little late because of a traffic jam.

He entered, grinning from ear to ear.

As they were having dinner, after Naresh had two drinks, he stood up.

"Kumar sir, you saved Kalwa. I forgave him because of you." Naresh was back to his usual bluff master self.

"Wait. There is some confusion. I thought Kalwa forgave you by taking his complaint back." Kumar looked at him perplexed.

"Sir, that's where you are wrong. After you left Kalwa's home, my brothers and their men visited him and forced him to sign that letter taking his complaint back. They were going to break his bones for the trouble he had caused me. But when he pleaded and said that Dr. Kumar had promised him that he won't have any trouble from our side, they left him. I forgave him to honor your words, sir. Or else we would have crushed him like an insect." Naresh thumped his foot on the ground to show how.

"Who Kalwa, what home, what promise!!" Kumar, Prem, and Lal wondered and looked at one another. They had made up a story to correct Naresh's bragging. But using that story as a foundation Naresh had built an even bigger lie!

"There is an old saying, you can't straighten the curved tail,... you know Kumar. Enjoy the beer while it's cold," Dr. Lal said picking up his mug. Naresh was still crushing the imaginary insect.

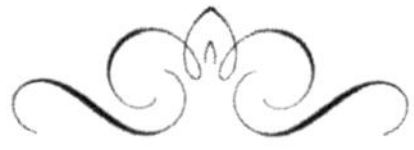

> The whole world is run on bluff.
>
> "Marcus garvey"

> After all, bluff and real emotion exist so easily side by side
>
> "Fyodor Dostoevsky"

A Greengrocer and Corona

"Have fresh green vegetables, have fresh fruits!"

The greengrocer kept calling as he pushed his cart full of vegetables and fruits through the narrow streets of Kutchesar village. Kutchesar was a typical Indian village with a mixed demography – a Hindu majority with a handful of Muslims, and both in turn divided into more castes and groups than the vegetables and fruits on the greengrocer's cart. What if the vegetables were Hindus and the fruits Muslim, or vice versa, he wondered. If there was a riot between the vegetables and fruits, who should he favor? If there was a crown king among vegetables, the brinjal, so was there one among the fruits, the mango.

"Have fresh beans, fresh cauliflowers, fresh spinach, onions, fresh carrots, fresh tomatoes, fresh potatoes, have coriander, have mint!" He called again.

But no one came to him. "Have fresh apples, fresh bananas, fresh oranges, fresh grapes!"

He was a regular sight in many of the nearby villages. Most were familiar with his voice and presence. They were used to him visiting after an intervals of three or four days. Women, with their children, would crowd around him. They especially enjoyed getting mint and coriander leaves complimentary with their purchases. But since the lockdown from March 24th, the streets had been deserted. Even he couldn't go selling his wares at first, till he got himself a curfew pass to visit each village once a week, and only on the condition he wore a mask and gloves, and kept his cart covered too as he moved. It was his first round to Kutchesar after a week.

He called once more... "Have fresh vegetables, have fresh fruits!"

But still no customers came. Why were people not coming, he wondered He checked his mask, it was in place; even his cart was well covered. His wife had torn an old, green chunni into two for this purpose – a small piece to cover his face and the rest to cover the cart. The green color matches the green vegetables, she thought.

He called yet once more, "Have green vegetables; have fresh fruits!"

Many people opened their doors, looked at him, and shut the doors again. I am coming after a week, so how could they still have enough stock, he asked himself. Maybe some other greengrocer has already visited recently before me? The street he was moving through was narrow and smoky. Some garbage had just been burnt. Burning garbage is a regular practice in almost all parts of India. Though much of the world had been pollution-free since the global lockdown, this street was still suffocating – courtesy the smoke. He decided to leave. The smoke was already making him cough.

"He is spreading corona," someone cried from a distance. "He is a Muslim, look at his green face cover."

"The mullah is coughing over the vegetables", a second harsh voice came. Till then he had been alone, but suddenly now many youngsters emerged with sticks, and started abusing him and beating him brutally.

"This is the agenda of Muslim Tabligi, they are spreading corona in Hindu areas by coughing or spitting over fruits and vegetables", someone in the group said.

"Yes, I have seen a video on WhatsApp. It showed a Muslim hairdresser in a salon spitting into the facial he was giving to a Hindu while the latter's eyes were closed", a second voice asserted.

"These are traitors, they are scoundrels", came a third voice. "Kill him."

The poor vegetable vendor tried to say something but failed. He tried to escape but fell down on the road with a large bleeding wound on his head. Trying hard to cover his head with both hands, he finally fainted. In the melee, the mask slipped partially off his face.

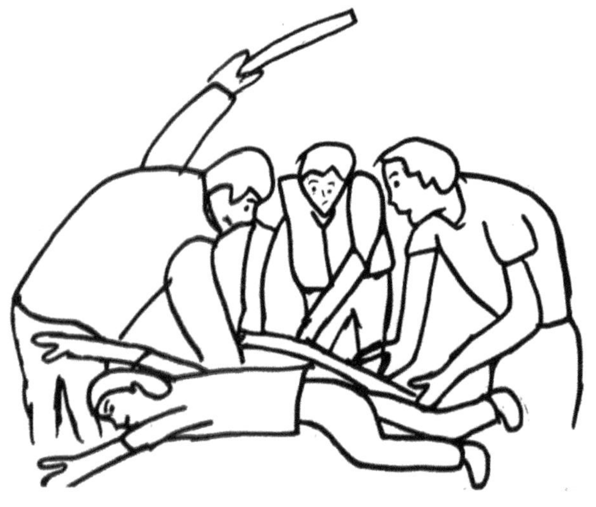

"He is Ramu, our regular vegetable vendor, someone cried. Aye stop, stop!"

They all stopped. Their hands, feet, and open mouths seemed to turn to stone.

"My God he is Ramu, our brother. We have sinned, even if it was by mistake. We could not identify him. He was wearing the green mask and we thought him a mullah. My God, he should have told us", someone said.

"Hey boys, hurry up, come on. Lift him; we have to take him to the doctor. We are short of time."

Five or six young men lifted the greengrocer up and took him to the only clinic in the village, which was run by Dr. Aleem But due to the lockdown, the clinic was closed.

One of the men who had hit Ramu with an iron rod ran to Dr. Aleem's residence close by and brought him to his clinic. Dr. Aleem gave Ramu first aid, stitched the wound, and dressed it.

"How did he get injured?" He asked.

The crowd felt ashamed. "Dr. Aleem, Bhai what to hide from you, actually we thought him a Tablighi Jamati spreading corona by coughing over his vegetables and fruits", one of them finally said.

"But he is Ramu. All of you know him. He has been coming here for years."

"Dr. Aleem, Bhai we could not recognize him, he was wearing a green mask and his voice seemed to be different too. There have been many viral videos claiming that Muslims are spreading corona across the country by different means. We had developed an irrational fear. My God, we would have killed one of our brothers today."

"But I am also a Muslim", said Dr. Aleem.

"No, you are our brother. We are truly ashamed. We all are brothers."

Ramu opened his eyes. "You people nearly killed me", he said. "Tell me my brothers, who is the brutal killer? Humans or the corona virus?" And he closed his eyes again, saying "Let's kill the hatred that divides our brotherhood."

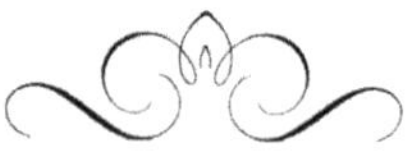

> Don't make me into this airy -fairy,moralist,idealist because I am not.
>
> "Madeleine albright"

A Mother and Her Son

Sumitra was chatting with other women of her village. One may wonder what women talk about when they are sitting together. They can talk for hours and maybe even days if they are not interrupted. Much of the discussion is often about the man they live with, but with whom they are never satisfied. They even say so at times to the men themselves. "It's only I who can put up with you. No other woman would stay with you. I am doing so for the sake of my parents. Otherwise, I would have fled." Yet on the day of *karwa chauth*, they fast for the longevity of their husbands and touch their feet too. They pray to be with the same worthless fool not only in their present life but in subsequent ones too.

Sumitra had run around for the blessings of every ulema, every sadhu-sanyasi, every tantrik whose name was suggested to her, in her efforts to conceive. She had knocked on every possible shrine's door. When she failed to conceive and gradually began ageing, someone suggested she try to have a test-tube baby. Her own patience, along with the hard work and experience of the medical team at the hospital she visited, finally enabled her to fulfill her dream. Thus was born her son Bablu, whom she considered her greatest strength. She pampered him with utmost care all through his childhood and beyond.

“Let him spend more time with his friends”, her husband Kishan suggested.

“I don't want another *lallu* or moron at home”, she answered. She never missed an opportunity to underscore to her husband that he was good for nothing. She would cite her son as a living example. Other than his birth your contribution to his growth is zero, zero and zero, she often chuckled.

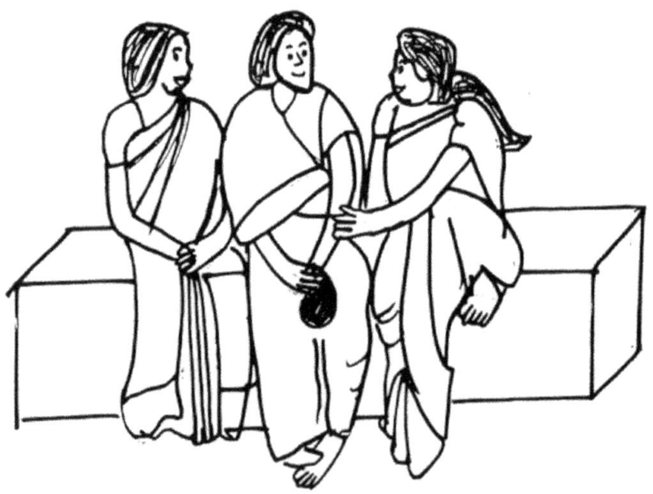

"My son is so gullible, so simple", she told her women friends as they chatted. She narrated an incident. "Once the chimney of a kerosene lamp they had in the house broke. The boy was asked to buy another one from the general store. He was so shy that at the shop, his soft mumble was hardly heard. When he asked for a 'chimney', the shopkeeper thought he wanted *chini* (sugar). It so happened that the shop didn't have *chini*, so the shopkeeper gave him *gur* (jaggery) instead. My sweet and simple boy brought home jaggery instead of a lamp chimney." All the women laughed till their chests hurt.

She ruled over Bablu like a dictator, enforcing strict discipline. But there was a volcano bubbling inside Bablu she remained unaware of.

Even after he had grown up and graduated, Bablu remained a teetotaler, thanks to his mother's dominance over him. His friends would tease him, asking him to go lie in his mother's lap and get himself breastfed.

Like the rest of the world, the locality Bablu and his parents lived in was also hit by Covid-19. It soon became a hotspot and strict lockdown was applied – Lockdown 1 moved on to Lockdowns 2, 3 and 4 stretching like the tail of Hanumanji before it began burning Lanka. Bablu and his parents remained stuck at home, hardly venturing out.

With time, however, essential items they had stocked were exhausted. Occasionally, Sumitra would give Bablu a bag and some cash and ask him to get rations from the nearby grocery store. Cash was already running short. "Sitting around with no work and earning nothing would have exhausted even Kuber's treasure hoard", said Sumitra. One day, just as she was sending Bablu out for rations, she began cursing her husband for being unemployed.

"Okay Ma, I'm leaving", Bablu replied and went out. But something was brewing in his mind.

Sumitra continued to curse. "For me to get work the market has to open again, and people have to come to the market", said her husband. "People are all at home because of the government order, my dear. It is the corona virus that is marching on roads and the markets are closed. It is the duty of the government to take care of us in this crisis." He too went away to play cards with his friends.

"Corona my foot, the government is also as good for nothing as you are", Sumitra said. "You are both using corona as a scapegoat."

....

Eight-nine hours later.

"My son is missing", shrieked Sumitra, beating her chest, shaking her husband who had long since returned home. "This is all because of you. You were good for nothing before and still you are the same."

"What happened to you?" He asked mildly.

"It's my bad luck to have such an irresponsible man as my husband."

"What's wrong with you Sumitra?" Her husband responded. "What wrong have I done other than marrying you?"

She had been screaming so loud that neighbors had started gathering hearing the noise.

"It's your fault. I kept him here for nine months", she said, patting her belly. "What did you do? You sent my son out during a lockdown to get rations." She put all the blame on him. "Are your legs broken that you couldn't go yourself? God knows where my son is. It's been hours since he went out and you are not worried at all. It was a mistake of my parents to marry me to you, such a useless man."

The neighbors asked her to calm down and file a complaint with the police. They all agreed it would be the best course. About to leave for the police station, Sumitra was locking her front door, her husband having already begun moving ahead, along with their neighbors, when suddenly she noticed a newly married couple coming towards her. They were both in wedding dress.

The boy looks familiar, she thought. The couple approached her and both bent down to touch her feet. Her husband and neighbors were also staring at the couple. The neighbors' whispering grew louder.

"Are you Bablu", she cried in amazement.

"Yes Ma", Bablu replied calmly.

"Who is she?"

"Ruchi, your bride, Ma."

"People everywhere are worrying about the deadly corona virus, and you were.........." She held her head in both her hands and sat down on the front porch.

"I was afraid of you, Ma."

"Did you know each other earlier?"

"Yes, Ma."

"For how long? Since when?"

"From the time you first sent me for rations. I met her at the shop."

"What about her family, her religion and caste?"

"Ma, a boy marries a girl – not her family, her religion or caste."

Sumitra was speechless suddenly. Bablu was no longer behaving like her son. The precious treasure she had kept for years was slipping away from her grasp.

"Have some shame. Everyone here is worrying about food during this time, while you..."

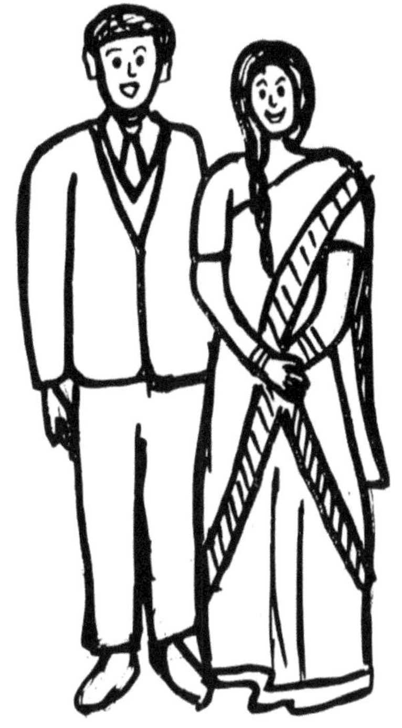

"He was worried about his bride, someone in the crowd said, to a burst of laughter."

"How could you think of that? She still could not believe it."

"Ma, corona is hitting more and more people worldwide and the aged are the most vulnerable. I thought if it picked you or Papa or both, your one desire would have remained unfulfilled. Many a times you said that you have only one desire left: to see my bride before closing your eyes forever."

"Have you married her?"

"Yes, Ma."

The dream fortress she had built and ruled over for years was shattered all of a sudden.

"I was a moron but not he", said her husband. "He is your son. He is smart enough to know how to butter his bread. The volcano you pampered underneath has erupted."

"And what about the rations I had asked you to buy?" Sumitra expressed her anger.

"She is herself a ration dealer, Ma. Now we will always have rations." Bablu smiled and sat at his mother's feet.

Sumitra looked at him. He may be a teetotaler, but he is also a fully grown man now, she realized.

She looked at her husband angrily. "Get some sweets", she said. "My son has come home with his bride."

"My husband is always useless," she said to Ruchi, the bride, and embraced her. She had smartly diverted the hurricane targeting her home.

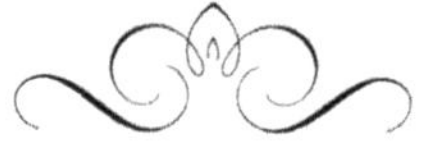

I hope the average woman feels she needs practicality with a little bit of fantasy. Otherwise, it's just not fashion.

"Francisco Costa"

Do it right or don't do it all . That comes from my mom.

"Ray Charles"

Delhi to Katihar

Laluwa sat in his Jhuggi (Slum dwelling) with two of his friends. All three were rickshaw wallahs working in different parts of Delhi. When Laluwa took the train from Katihar to Delhi 12 years ago, this wasn't the future he had expected.

He was the eldest of four brothers and two sisters. They lived in a mud house in Katihar. It was the only inheritance his father had received from his grandfather, along with a debt of Rs 200 when his grandfather died. He and his siblings all attended primary school just for the mid-day meal they got there, the only meal they could be sure of.

As Laluwa grew older, his family's poverty became intolerable to him. He wanted to get out of this state. Many times, he had expressed his wish to go to a big city, where he believed there were better opportunities of finding employment. At least he would be able to provide for his younger siblings. But his father, the simple man he was, never approved of it. He thought of cities as demons that devoured people like him and his family and spat out their carcasses. In the village, they were poor but at least they were together. The difference in father and son's viewpoints increased with time, and one day when the gap became too large to hold them together, Laluwa left for the city against his father's will.

Laluwa had heard many stories of how people had transformed their destinies in Delhi. He too wanted his own rags to riches story. Brimming with hope and young blood in his veins, he had boarded the train to Delhi. But his dreams were quashed on the city's roads. The blinding light of the city took away the shine of his eyes. His youthful energy was drained by the city's fast tempo.

Laluwa remembered the day he was leaving for the city. His mother had offered him roti.

With his hand outstretched he took the roti and said "*Ma, aisi roti shehar mein nahi milegi* (Mother, I won't get such food in the city.)

Laluwa must have dozed off and spoken out loud because he suddenly felt some water being sprinkled on him. "Are you dreaming," he heard his friend Madhav say. "We have not had roti for two days."

Laluwa was soon fully awake. As he stretched and yawned, he felt a sharp pain in his elbow.

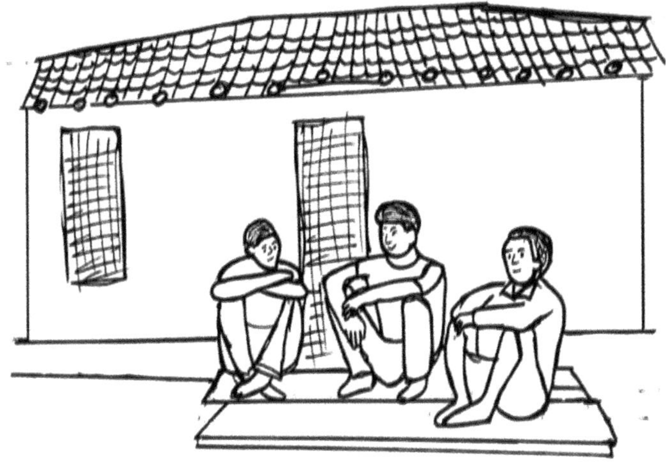

He remembered how he had got the bruises on his hand and back. It was at the roadside the previous day while trying to get food.

He remembered the prime minister addressing the nation a week back. "There will be three weeks of complete lockdown to counter the threat of the corona pandemic. The whole world is terrified. It's for you, my dear countrymen, for the safety of your life that this lockdown is being imposed."

Yes, the safety of life is above everything else. Once the lockdown began, they were unable to get any work. Whatever rations they had were gradually consumed. Their neighbors' condition was no different from theirs. None of them earned enough to think of saving for themselves. All of them sent home whatever surplus funds they acquired. Laluwa too had sent money to his father a little before Holi just three weeks ago. He hadn't kept back much for himself thinking he would earn well during the festival, as many people went visiting at the time. "So what if we aren't able to go home for the festival, at least our families will celebrate well with the money we send them," Laluwa had thought. Now he was seriously short of cash. The rent for their *jhuggi* was also pending. The landlord could visit any day, and if they were not able to pay the rent, he would have their belongings thrown out on the road. Laluwa checked his pockets and found just one hundred rupee note and some change.

The three men again went out in search of food and returned with more bruises – both from the police for violating the lockdown, and some due to fights that broke out while they were trying to get food at relief centers. Madhav was the only one who managed to grab a packed meal. He brought it back to their room to share with the others. Even in such a situation, he couldn't imagine eating it alone. He would never compromise his friendship with the other two for just a meal.

They shared the meal and drank a lot of water to make up for the lack of solid food. Each one wrapped a long piece of cloth tightly around their stomach. It was a trick to reduce the pangs of hunger that poverty had taught them. They comforted each other and tried to sleep. Laluwa, in his slumber, could hear the continuous whistle of a railway engine passing nearby. "No trains are running in the lockdown; I must be dreaming," he thought. He saw a child riding on a slowly speeding train.

...

When Laluwa came to Delhi, travelling ticket less on the roof of the Mahananda Express, he was just 12 years old.

In his initial days in the big city, he stayed with one of his distant relatives in a slum. For a person coming from a small village to a metro, everyone hailing from his village is like a distant relative. Initially, he worked – as a waiter in a local food stall and as a helper to a motor mechanic. After some time, he finally managed to get a rickshaw to drive paying a daily rent. "That's where the money is," he thought. “If you work extra hours at night, you are allowed to charge passengers more. You can make much more money with a fewer number of rides.” He learnt from experience that the most generous passengers were young, unmarried couples and foreigners. They never bargained; on the contrary, they often paid a little more than the regular fare. Soon Laluwa had saved enough to buy his own rickshaw in partnership with his friend, Madhav. The rickshaw was used 24/7 as they both drove it in separate shifts. Life was good.

“The lockdown is going to be extended for a month or may be even two!!” The news spread through the slum faster than the virus.

"Corona might not kill us, but this hunger surely will," said Madhav. “A slow death by starvation would be much more painful than dying from an unknown disease.”

They went to sleep with these thoughts.

....

Next morning:

“Wake up Laluwa. Wake up. We are going home,” Madhav said.

“When? How?” Laluwa wasn't sure if he was dreaming again.

“The government has arranged buses at the Anand Vihar bus station to take people back home if they want to leave.”

The only valuable they possessed was their rickshaw. Planning to park it at the rickshaw stand close to the bus station before catching the bus home, they set off in the rickshaw.

They found hundreds of people on the road with a similar purpose, all on their way to the bus stand. Near Anand Vihar, they found the roads, deserted till the previous day, now chockablock with people. From hundreds, the number rose to thousands the closer they got to the bus stand.

Laluwa saw an unending line of heads waiting in lines to enter the buses.

As they parked their rickshaw and joined one of the queues, they spoke to an elderly person in the line ahead of them. He was mumbling. "It's happening again," he said. "I saw this when I was 10 years old, in 1947, at the time of Partition. Millions of people were going to Pakistan; millions were coming from Pakistan and millions died on the way. Now, 85 years old, I'm seeing it again. Are we not in our own country? Is there to be more division?"

They spent hours at the bus station, as the sun traveled and changed color from its subtle orange at dawn to a burning yellow. The hopes of those who had queued up faded and turned to agony as the queues did not move at all. At last, the officials at the bus station announced that due to some miscommunication among different state administrations, no buses could be arranged that day.

What!!! Laluwa and Madhav were appalled.

"Isn't what we are going through already bad enough that you had to play this cruel joke on us!" some people shouted, while some others broke down in despair.

"What do we do now?" Laluwa sat down on the road where he had been standing. His eyes welled up with tears.

"I can't take it. This is not fair. I gave my blood and sweat to this city and this is how it treats us? I want to go home. I have to get back home," he heard Madhav yelling in frustration.

Hope is a strange thing. Laluwa briefly lost it completely. But soon the hope of seeing his family again filled him with a new energy.

"Yes, we have to go home. And nobody can stop us." Laluwa got back on his feet with newfound determination. Maybe when one touches rock bottom, the only direction left to go is upwards.

"But how will we go home? It's more than 1,400 kms away," Madhav asked.

"With the only thing that we have – our rickshaw," said Laluwa, as he hurried towards the rickshaw parking stand.

They started their journey, pedaling in shifts. Fortunately, they found some kind people distributing biscuits, fruits and water bottles free near the bus station. Consuming whatever they could get, they felt God himself was blessing their journey. Even Madhav's spirit rekindled.

On their journey, they saw many even less fortunate than themselves, whole families who had set out on similar journeys on foot, some carrying small children on their shoulders. "We are not alone," Laluwa thought. They were lucky they had their rickshaw.

With every push of the rickshaw pedal, they knew they were getting closer to home. After pedaling for three hours straight, they stopped to drink water. Later, at another place, they saw tea and biscuits being distributed free. They stopped; the tea felt like a luxury.

They moved on. They saw policemen on the roads in certain places distributing free food and water. This was one aspect of the police, whom they mostly feared and avoided, they had never seen before. One police officer even smiled at them and wished them luck on the journey ahead. This virus had surely changed the world.

They stopped at Aligarh, having covered more than 150 kms from Delhi, to rest. While passing though Prayagraj, another 500 kms eastwards, they paid obeisance to the holy river Ganga. "O mother Ganga, save us and all our country from this calamity," they prayed.

Twelve days after they left Delhi, they reached their destination, their home, Katihar. The sturdy rickshaw had not let them down.

When Laluwa entered his home, his mother hugged him. Her love took away all the fatigue of the journey.

After a few minutes, she broke the embrace and asked him, "You must be hungry. Did you find something to eat on the way?"

"It was a long journey Ma, a long journey ....of .....12 days," he said.

"12 days? ......You've been away 12 years, yes, it was a long journey back, my son," his father said, smiling from where he sat, in a corner of their half brick and half mud house.

His younger sister brought him warm milk and sattu. "You must be tired and aching all over, bhaiya," she said, touching his arm.

The healed bruises Laluwa had received while hunting for food in Delhi began to hurt severely again. His tears fell freely. At least at home I am not going to die of hunger, as a destitute, he thought. It was better to live with broken dreams than to lose one's life.

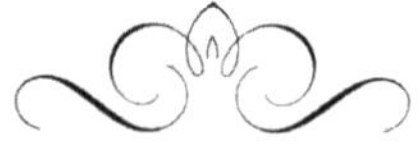

> An imbalance between rich and poor is the oldest and most fatal ailment of all republics.
>
> "Pluto parch"

Who Killed Him?

Even the Spanish flu of a century ago did not achieve the notoriety Covid-19 has. The Spanish flu claimed 50 million lives worldwide, but, unlike with Covid-19, there remained some countries it did not touch. In the destruction and pain it has inflicted, Covid-19 is by far the greatest tragedy the world has faced after World War II.

At the height of the lockdowns governments imposed to contain Covid-19, roads became deserted, people stayed indoors, and mothers hid their children fearing the virus would infect them. It remains the adversary. No single development before had made people panic, the way Covid-19 has. The world is cursing China for creating the monster. China is accusing America of being the perpetrator. Two of the most powerful nations on earth are quarreling like the parents of a spoiled son and blaming each other, neither willing to own him. Crawling in the lap of mother China and hitting so-called father America on the head (China has contained the virus, while in the US, deaths are still mounting heavily), Covid-19 has turned into a Bhasmasur. Bhasmasur was the demon in an indian epic story where after getting the boon that he can kill anyone placing his hand over their head, from lord Shiva the demon ran behind to kill his creator.

In India, all the fighting is internal. Though they are all rooted in the same soil, the people of Aryavarta have followed different faiths. Though they grew on the same land, nourished by the same sun, they keep finding small things to quarrel over. "Your forefathers abused mine" or “God has authorized us to rule” are good enough for one group to attack another.

Amar and Abdul worked in Surat in a textile unit. Both hailed from Ayodhya - the town of Lord Ram – 1,400 kms to the northeast. Lord Ram, when he lived, had set the example of how an ideal man should act. His kingdom was believed to have been an abode of justice and abundance for all.

Surat is in Gujarat - a textile hub and world renowned for its diamond polishing industry. With the nationwide lockdown, all the industries in Surat were also closed. Like thousands of others, Amar and Abdul too had come to Surat seeking food and shelter. With the lockdown stretching for months, they did not need an astrologer to foretell their future. "We have to live with corona," the statement of India’s prime minister and other global leaders was ringing in their ears.

"The lockdown is like the endless tail of Hanumanji in Lanka, destroying everything," said Amar.

"It's already been over two months without work." Abdul looked serious.

"The world has to live with corona, Abdul. That's what people are saying."

"Yes, but how will we live without work? It looks like we are becoming a social liability now."

"How?" asked Amar.

"We have been surviving on Government grants and our employer's generosity. I feel it's disgraceful. We are losing our self-respect day by day."

"I think you are right, Abdul."

"We are not beggars! We are artisans. We live off the sweat of our brow. Day by day, we are losing our dignity, Amar."

Amar had a bout of coughing. Abdul gave him a glass of water. They were childhood friends, working in the same factory and had been living together since they came to Surat. They were more like brothers than friends. They shared the same kind of brotherhood Rama and Laxman had shown the world ages ago.

Amar looked a little uncomfortable.

"Sorry, Amar, if I hurt you. But it's obvious which way the wind will blow in coming days."

"You are correct. But what option do we have?"

"Amar, I heard many of our fellow workers are going back to their villages. Even our employers are getting financially exhausted and may not support us much longer... Our needs are minimal back in our villages."

Amar could see the resolution in Abdul's eyes.

Along with some other workers, they decided to go back home the very next day. One of the senior workers booked a truck, and Amar and Abdul started their journey back to Ayodhya. They were forty-five of them adjusted somehow in the limited space at the back of the truck. They travelled via Vadodara, Ujjain and Guna.

Soon, they were just a day away from reaching Ayodhya. "We are moving fast, will arrive earlier than we expected," Amar said. "There is hardly any traffic on the road. It looks like a river and we alone are ruling it."

They saw a few other groups of laborers too, who were making their way home on foot.

Ujjain is well known for its Mahakaleshwar Temple. As their truck passed it, they all joined their palms and prayed to the Lord to have mercy on them. Abdul too followed their example. They stopped briefly for a meal arranged for them by the local police and residents.

Abdul didn't eat his packed meal but kept it for later.

"I will have it in the evening, after my roza", he said. It was the month of Ramadan and he was fasting. It was only then that reminded the others he was a Muslim.

The truck began moving again. Suddenly one of the workers shouted out, looking at Abdul: "Because of you people, we are all suffering."

Abdul was not at all ready for this attack. He was on the 20th day of his Ramadan fast, and feeling rather weak. He decided not to respond.

"After pushing the whole country into a disaster, you are fasting and will enjoy Eid too," his heckler added.

"What rubbish are you saying?" Amar responded, simmering with anger. Abdul still remained cool.

"Yes, the corona virus has been spread by the Muslim Tablighi." Someone else among the workers spoke up.

They had been ordinary workers a few minutes ago. Suddenly, a few of them now became Hindus first. Abdul was turned into a Tablighi with a corona stamp.

"You've known me for a long time. I am neither a Tablighi nor a jamaati. I am your brother," Abdul replied calmly. "Tablighis were victims of the corona virus too, like many others. Corona has no religion."

A heated discussion followed. Abdul pointed out that while the Tablighi Jamaat, which had gone ahead with its meeting in the early days of the lockdown, and might have inadvertently spread the corona virus, could be held guilty to some extent, it had not created the virus. "Look at Wuhan, China where this monster struck first, look at Italy and the rest of the western world," he said. "There is no Jamaat there, but all these countries are suffering. Look at America, which has had so many deaths. The whole world is under the cruel paw of this monster. Yes, those Jamaatis who were responsible for the meeting will face the consequences."

Amar had begun to feel dryness in his throat. He was unhappy with this turn of the conversation. He had been coughing earlier; he had another bout of cough. Abdul gave him some water; he drank it.

"This is a disease caused by that evil virus," Amar said. "The virus is not going to spare Muslim or Hindu. The Christian nations have already been devastated. We need to hate the virus, not each other." He had yet another coughing fit. He felt weak.

He has fever, someone said. All became concerned. Was it Covid-19 he was suffering from? The truck had just passed Guna. They tried to sit as far away from Amar as possible. Only Abdul remained next to Amar, giving him water to drink and repeatedly trying to cool his forehead with his wet hanky.

He has corona, the same man shouted again. He asked the driver to stop immediately. He wanted Amar out of the truck. Abdul requested the others to wait until the truck reached the next town, Shivpuri, where Amar and he would voluntarily leave. "Don't drop us here in the middle of the highway with no transport in sight," he pleaded. But all his requests were in vain. Amar was offloaded in the middle of nowhere by his own religious brothers. All Abdul could do was also step out of the truck with Amar.

While they had been aboard the truck, the deserted roads had looked beautiful. Now the same empty road looked frightening. For hours, Abdul could find no conveyance to travel further, while Amar still burnt with fever. He wearily sat down on the shoulder of the road with Amar's head in his lap. He wept. Amar was unconscious now. The nearest hospital was miles away in Shivpuri.

Abdul raised his eyes as he heard the sound of a three-wheeler. Yes indeed, an empty three-wheeler was passing by. "Something wrong," the driver asked.

Unable to answer, Abdul still sobbed. The driver stopped and stepped out. He touched Amar's forehead.

"My God, he has high fever," the driver muttered. "He is unconscious too." Abdul and he lifted Amar and laid him on the passenger seat of the three-wheeler. The driver gave full throttle to the engine. He wanted to reach Shivpuri, and find a hospital there, as quickly as possible. But it took time. Shivpuri was forty miles away. The three-wheeler raced. For Abdul, every minute was like a yug, a millennium. Reaching the hospital, the driver and he rushed Amar to the casualty department.

The doctor on duty examined Amar. Looking serious, he asked if an ECG had been taken.

"Sir, the ECG is flat," said his assistant, showing it to him. "Who is he to you?" The doctor asked Abdul.

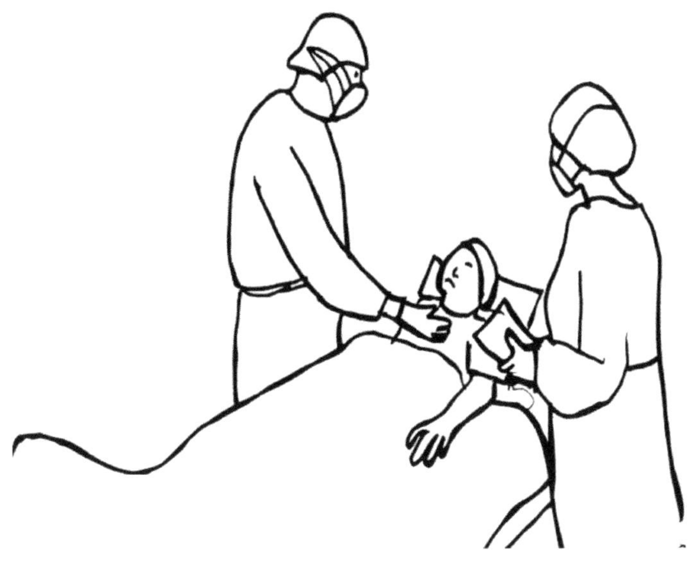

"He is my brother," Abdul replied. "Save him, doctor." He sat down on the floor, bent.

"Sorry, he is no more," said the doctor.

"Means?"

"He is dead," the doctor said raising Abdul from the floor.

Amar lay on the stretcher. Abdul stood by his side holding his hand. His eyes were red. Mentally, he sought an explanation from God. Who killed Amar? Was it the corona virus or fear of the corona virus... or his religious Hindu brothers who left him in the wilderness, or ...the Tablighi jamaatis, who are blamed for spreading corona in the country?

Only Abdul had stood by Amar like Laxman – the true brother of Lord Rama.

> Love is the only force capable of transforming an enemy into a friend .
>
> "Martin Luther King, Jr"

Just a day of Quarantine

"Sir, her COVID -19 test is positive."

"Whose?" I asked!

"That patient's, Aarifa."

I eyed Bablu. It was as if he had exploded a bomb on my head. I had operated on Aarifa three days ago. She had slipped and fallen down the stairs; her spleen had been shattered. Her abdomen was full of blood. She was in shock and had to be attended to immediately.

Bablu was our staff-in-charge. The Covid-19 test is mandatory for patients coming to the hospital from high-risk hotspot Covid areas. The test was carried out, her nasal and throat swabs sent to the lab, but the report would take 48 hours. There was no time to wait for it. We decided to save the patient.

"Aarifa's Covid-19 test report had been positive", he repeated.

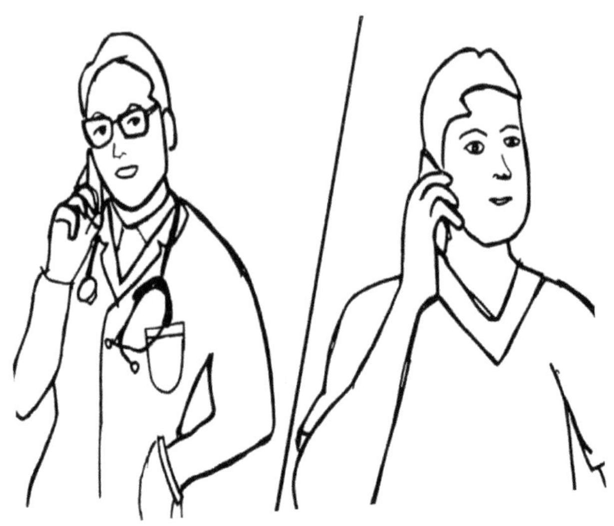

"Hun...", I just shook my head.

His words were like melted hot glass poured into my ears. Both my feet felt frozen. The patient had been asymptomatic, with nothing about her suggesting she had the virus. In the last two months of Lockdown we had done dozens of emergency surgeries like hers, carrying out a routine Covid-19 test each time whose result always came two days later. In all such previous cases, the corona test results had been negative. A deadly snake seemed to be tightening its coils around my neck, preparing to bite. We had taken every routine precaution during the surgery, but we knew there might have been many lacunae.

The whole team would have to be quarantined. The tea I was having tasted bitter in my mouth.

The District Administration was informed. A team of health officials from the District Chief Medical Officer's (CMO) department soon descended on our hospital. The operation theatre where the patient had undergone the surgery, the ICU, where she had been briefly kept after surgery, and the room she had stayed in, were sanitized again and locked for 24 hrs. The patient was sent off by ambulance to the nearest Covid-19 hospital. A list of doctors, operation theatre staff, ICU and other staff, was made and handed over to the CMO's office.

The first to attend to the patient and give her first aid had been Dr. Vinita. She lived in a joint family at Indralok, a posh colony. She had tears in her eyes; her only son was hardly five years old. Her heart was full of emotions for her son, her husband and others in her family. She rang her husband, who informed the other family members. He advised the obvious – "she should stay in hospital, and away from the family, till her quarantine period ended." She felt like Sita in the Ramayana being banished from Ayodhya by Lord Rama.

The second in the list of those being quarantined was the staff nurse who had taken the patient's blood sample and given her initial treatment. Anjali was always jolly. She was unmarried and came from a very poor family. "So what if the patient's report is positive, I am a corona girl now and I pledge to marry a man who will wear the crown of corona", she said laughing. She laughed till her chest started to hurt. "I will sketch a beautiful portrait of you, in isolation", she said to me. "It will be a good opportunity to rest and to draw". Her family, as well as the financial and social challenges she had faced and overcome, gave her the strength she showed.

The third to have attended to the patient was the anesthetist, a retired army Major, Dr. Sandeep Shekhar. He had served in the army medical corps for more than ten years, but had since become a freelance anesthetist. He had intubated the patient through the oral route and had continuously sat next to her, monitoring her throughout the operation. He laughed on hearing the test result. "At least half the corona viruses she exhaled must have gone into me", he said. An anesthetist has to sit close to the patient's mouth. He decided to take two large pegs of Goan feni with hot water. "Let the virus get confused and sink into the feni, it's purely Indian, neither Chinese nor American", he said. He decided that he and I would quarantine in the same room.

"You, I and feni will be gloriously quarantined", he said. "Relax Honey". He always called me 'Honey'. I wanted to laugh but could not bring myself to.

The fourth person who had interacted with the patient had been me. I started estimating the number of days I would have to be quarantined. On the fifth day from our exposure, we would have to send our throat and nasal samples to the lab, and then again on the tenth day. If both samples proved negative, the quarantine would end, but if one of them turned out positive ....I could already visualize Yama on his buffalo coming towards me.

I closed my eyes. I prepared a document listing my insurance policies, my assets and liabilities. I silently thanked the insurance agent who had badgered me into taking a life insurance policy for Rs 1 crore (Ten Million). I was sure my wife would get the money and would thus be financially secure, even if corona was not merciful to me. For the first time in my married life of 22 years I felt a deep love for my wife. She had served me and stood by me like a rock in all the ups and downs of my life. She had served my parents too untiringly. She was hardly 50, and could even consider remarrying. I felt deeply for her. I wanted to hug her. But corona had now made it impossible, even if we met. On the financial side, thankfully, I found that my liabilities were much less than my assets. I saw no reason to worry for my children. They were already grown up.

There were also my two OT assistants who would be quarantined. Aleem and Arun were quite happy about it. We would like to stay someplace close to you, sir, one of them said. Arun was angry with the corona virus. Belonging to a poor family, he had sacrificed much to make his other family members secure. His younger brother and sisters had married before him. At the age of forty, he found himself alone and finally decided to wed. His wedding had been fixed for April, but by then the first and second lockdowns had been enforced, and it had to be postponed. "I will cut corona into pieces with this surgical knife", he said.

Aleem was the optimistic kind. "God has given life and HE will decide the length of our lives too", he said. He turned to me. "You are our teacher, sir, we did what we were supposed to do", he added. "To save someone's life is more important than going for the Haj to Mecca." Many times he would even skip namaz if there was work to do at the hospital. "Sir, work is worship", he said.

"YOU are becoming a philosopher now", I said. He had made me relax. I smiled. "Yes in the Bhagwad Geeta, Lord Krishna said, we all should do our work. Rest we should leave to HIM". I uttered fully agreeing with him.

Two more who would face the same fate were our ICU and nursing staffers, Sandeep and Anshika. Both were true warriors. "Sir, the army fights the enemy at our borders", Anshika said. "Our great soldiers have done it from time to time and again and again. Now there is this invisible enemy that is inside our country and we medical staff are the soldiers who have to fight it. It's our turn now. So what if the enemy is invisible, so what if we have logistical shortcomings. We are not going to give up. Our morale is high and we will win this war." Anshika was half Hindu and half Christian. Her full name was Anshika Nelson.

"If we do not fight it, who else will sir", Sandeep said. He was the introverted sort. But he was clear in his thoughts and deeds.

The last two to be quarantined were Asha and Savitri, our housekeeping staff. They kept the beds and the floors clean, and carried out other duties no one else would. "We have nothing to lose, sir", said Asha. "Our life is a burden. What do we lose if corona takes us away?" They laughed. "Sir, even corona will not be able to bear visiting us", one of them added. "We will be grateful to corona if it relieves us of this disgraceful life."

I was speechless.

The Covid-19 positive patient was taken to the Covid hospital and her whole family was quarantined. The family members' throat and nasal samples were sent to the lab.

The top floor of our hospital was set aside for those quarantined. Dr. Sandeep Shekhar and I stayed in one room, and the others in different rooms. I did go home once, in my car, but only up to the gate. My own home, my wife, my kids all looked like strangers to me. They gazed at me from a long distance, with the closed gate of my house between us. Hardcore criminals are kept behind iron bars, and now there were iron bars separating me from my family.

My wife had packed lunch for me in a lunchbox, which she hung on a hook on our gate. Before I could open the gate, she had retreated. I could not get the lunch, as a big monkey appeared out of nowhere and made off with the lunchbox. I phoned my wife using my mobile. She was merciful and brought a second lunchbox, this time with Tyson, our Labrador, escorting her. She ordered from a distance, to open the gate. Without a word I took the lunchbox and had my lunch. I hung the empty lunchbox on the gate.

In the evening, Dr. Sandeep Shekhar said to me, "relax Honey, take it easy." He brought out a pack of cards and we decided to play bluff. In every relationship of life, there is some bluffing involved. Corona had made that clear. Shekhar made large pegs of feni. We both drank.

"It smells of cashew", I said. I was tasting it for the first time.

"Yes, it's a cashew drink. Honey, think we are in Goa", he said.

We drank four Patiala pegs of feni and dreamed of roaming on beautiful Goa beaches as we slept.

Someone was knocking on the door.

Who is disturbing us in Goa, was my first thought. The mobile phone was also continuously ringing. I put the phone on silent mode. Again someone knocked even more forcibly on the door.

Stop, coming brother, don't break the door, I said sleepily. I opened it. To my surprise, my wife was in front of me, my children and Tyson too with her. There was bright sunshine outside the window. I had overslept.

"When did you come to GOA? I asked." I was confused, still rubbing my eyes.

"You are not in Goa, you are here in Haripur", she said. Pinching my cheeks, she hugged me tightly. In bits and pieces came the explanation. The patient Arifa's report and those of her family members had turned out to be negative. The first lab had given a faulty report. My quarantine was over. Our CMO had been trying to call me for a long time but I had not answered his calls. I had been dreaming of roaming in Goa. Failing to speak to me, the CMO informed my wife.

She looked so happy. Unable to control her emotions, she started kissing me. I looked at my children and at Dr. Sandeep Shekhar. He was still sleeping. The kids were happy as their mother. They too hugged me, their eyes speaking volumes. "WE WILL NOT LET YOU GO, PAPA", they said. Tyson was wagging his tail like a fan and was trying to climb on top of me. At a distance, I could see Yama on his black buffalo retreating, tired and disappointed.

The only thing we have to fear is fear itself.

"Franklin D. Rooseevelt"

www.ingramcontent.com/pod-product-compliance
Ingram Content Group UK Ltd.
Pitfield, Milton Keynes, MK11 3LW, UK
UKHW021658190726
13853UKWH00001B/337